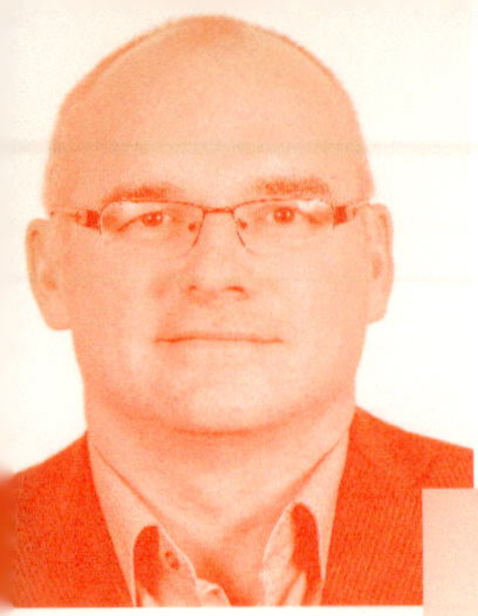
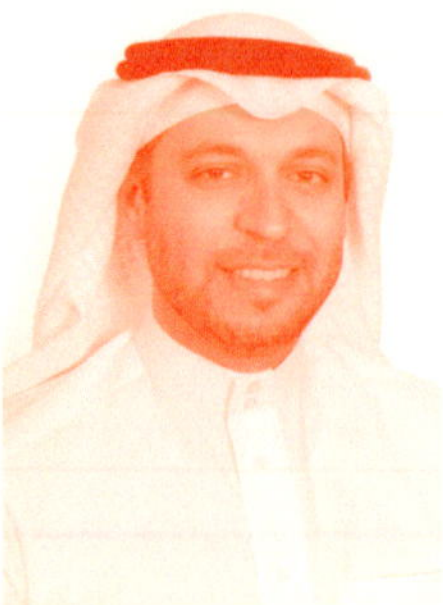
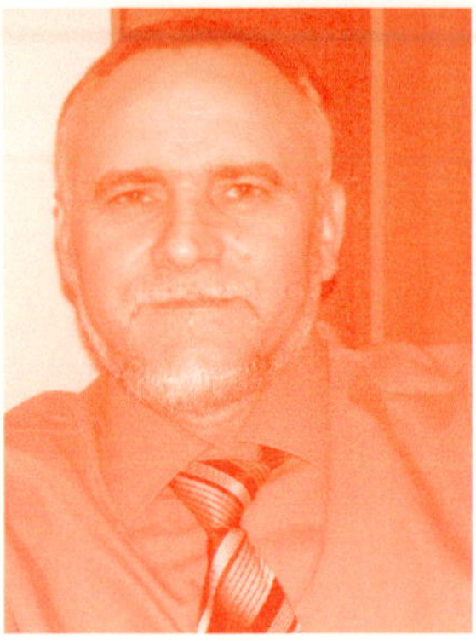
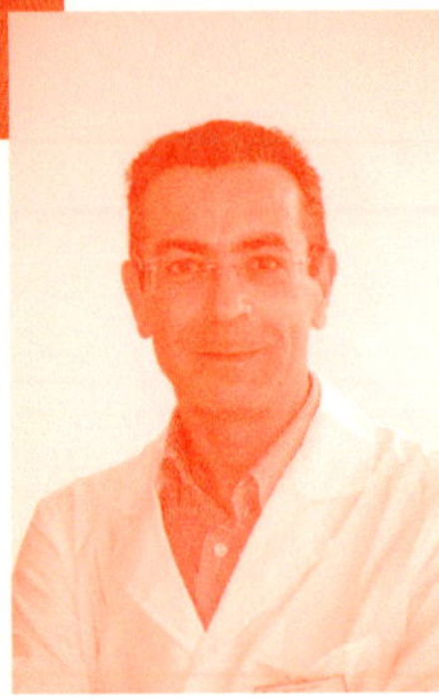
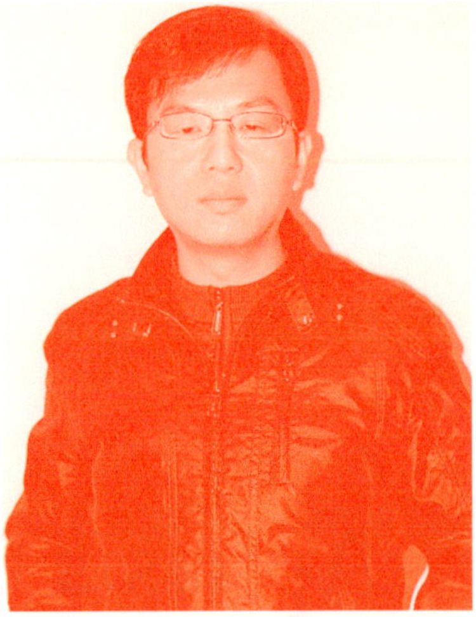
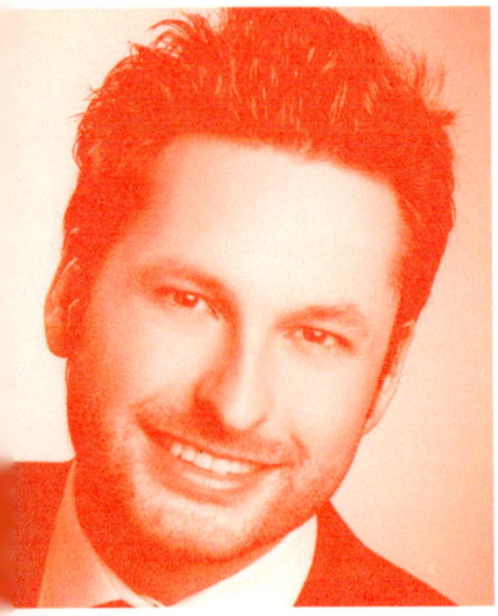
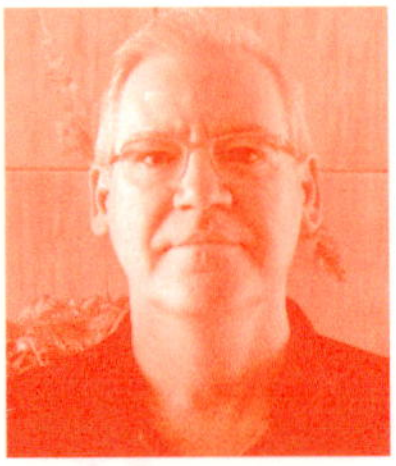

IntechOpen

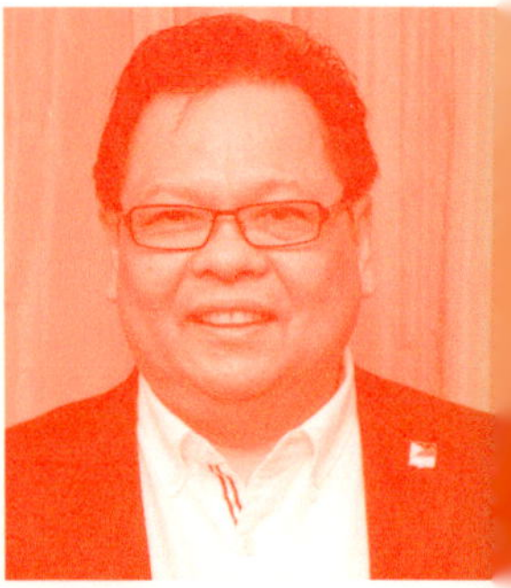
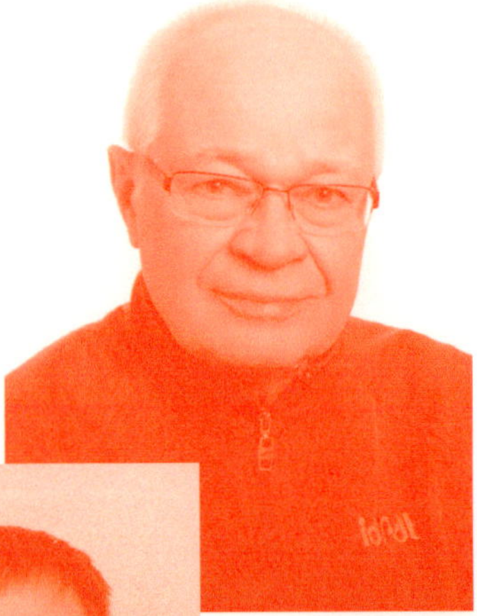
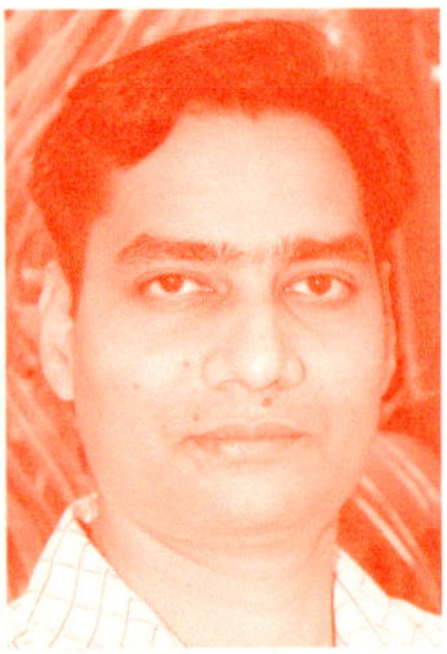
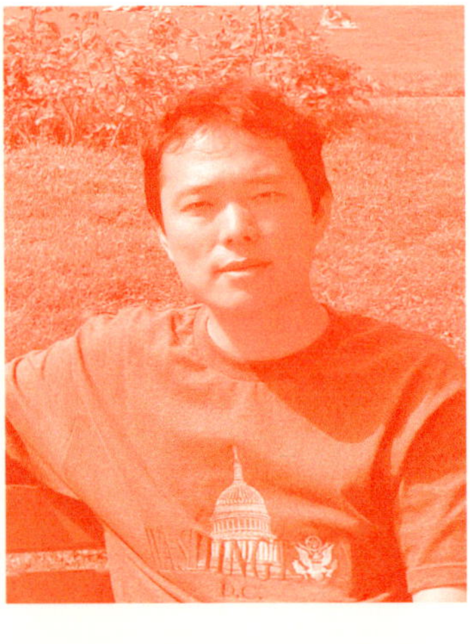
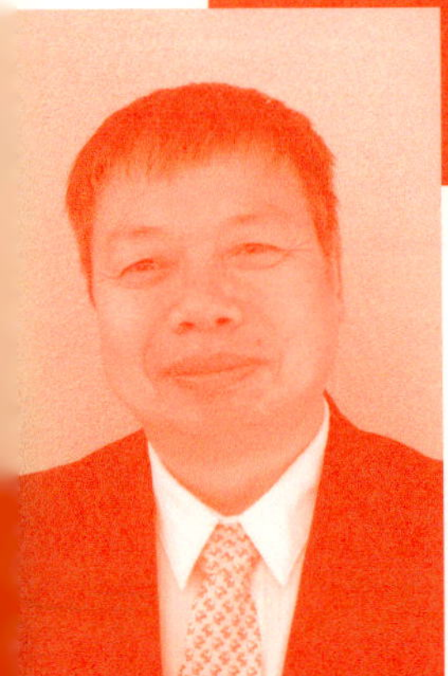
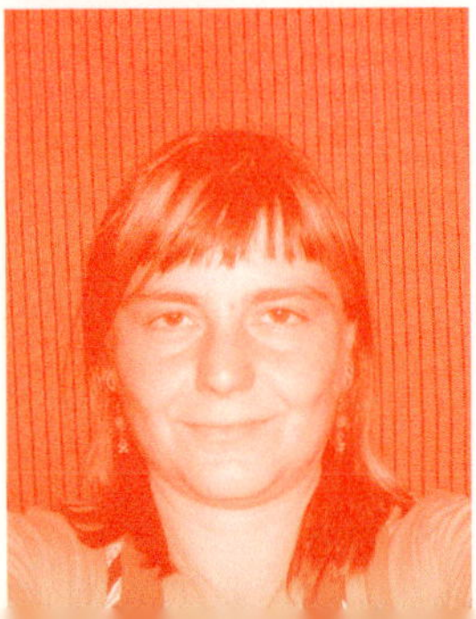

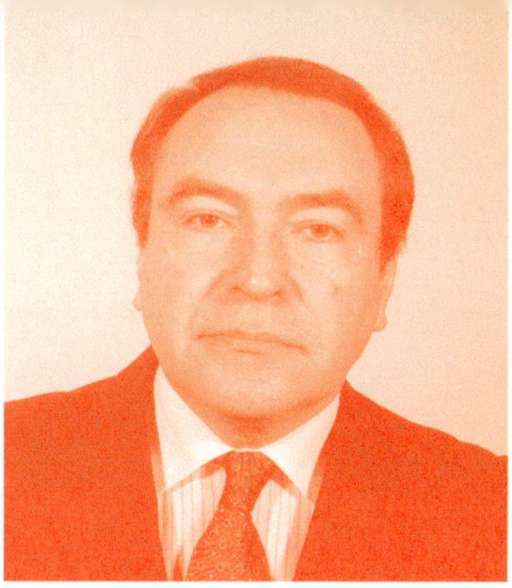
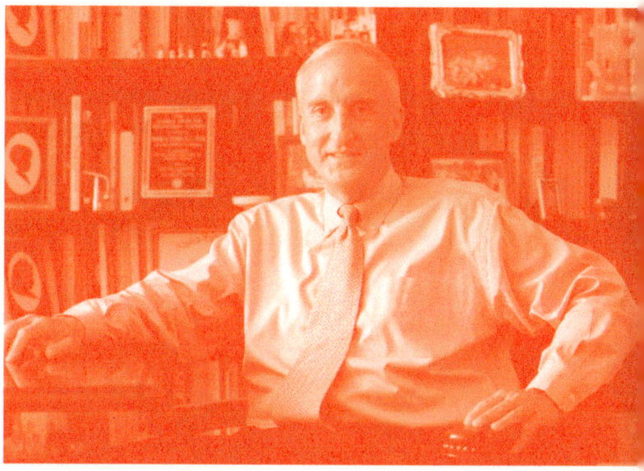
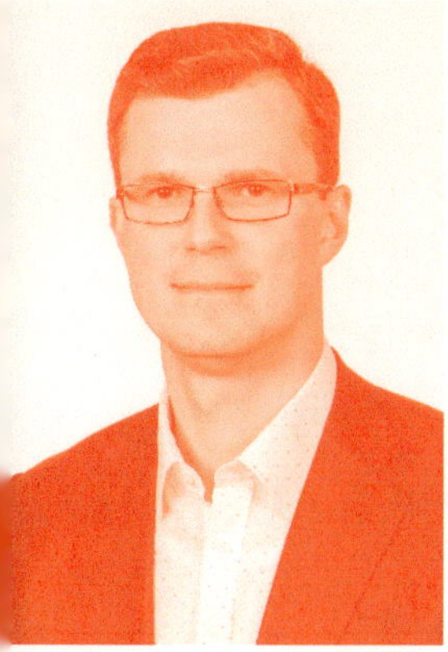
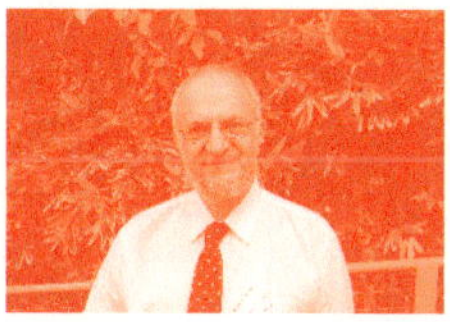
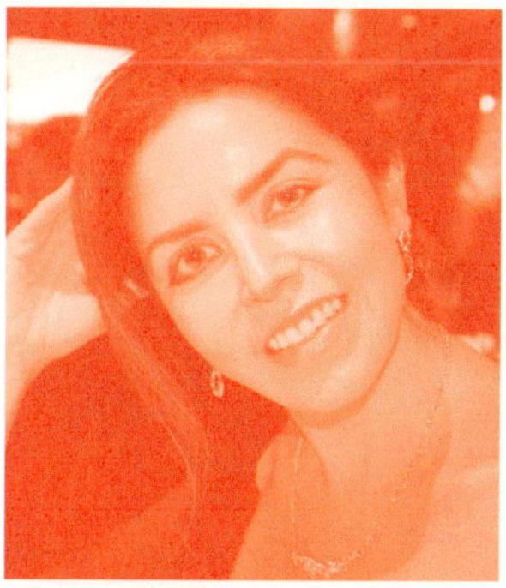

Supporting open minds since 2005

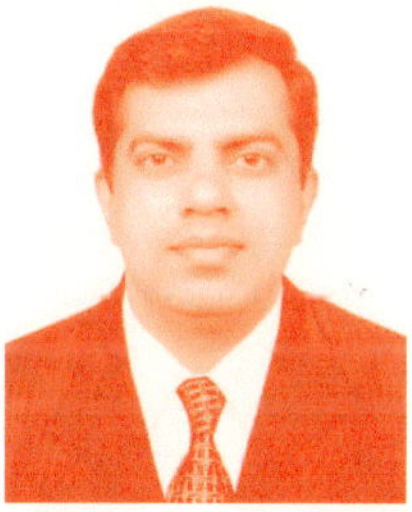
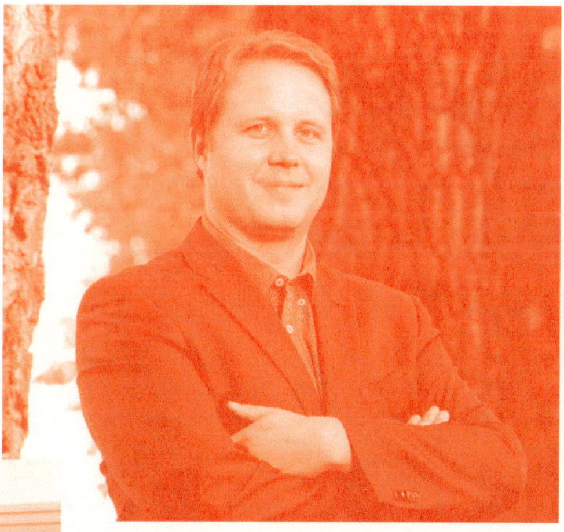
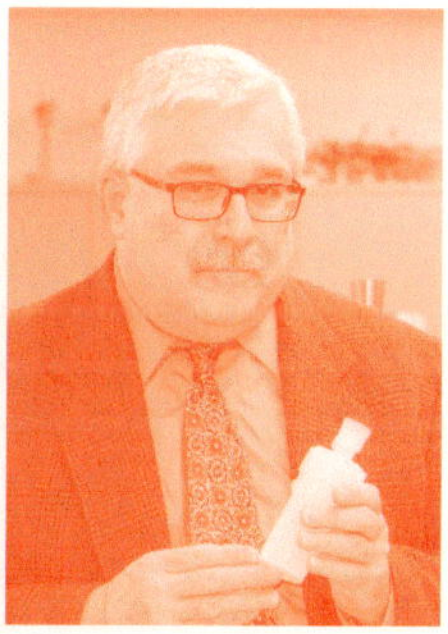
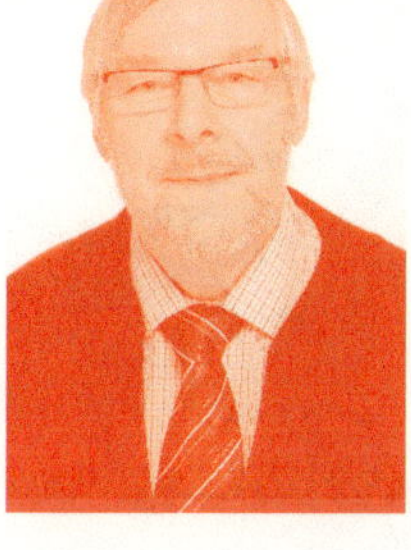
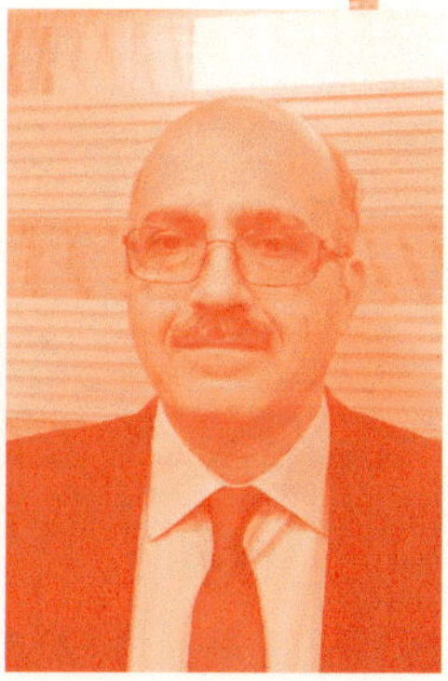
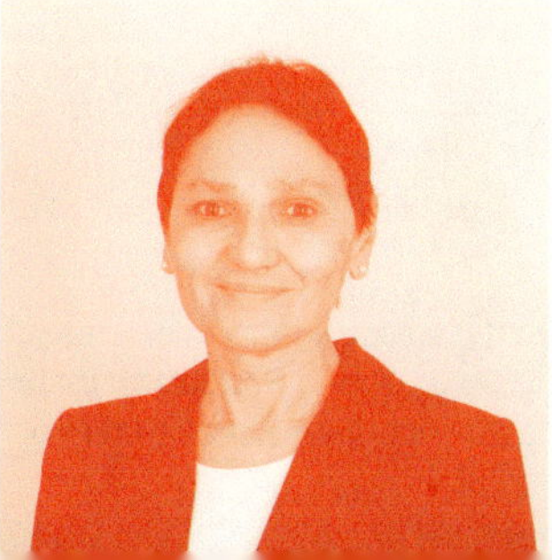
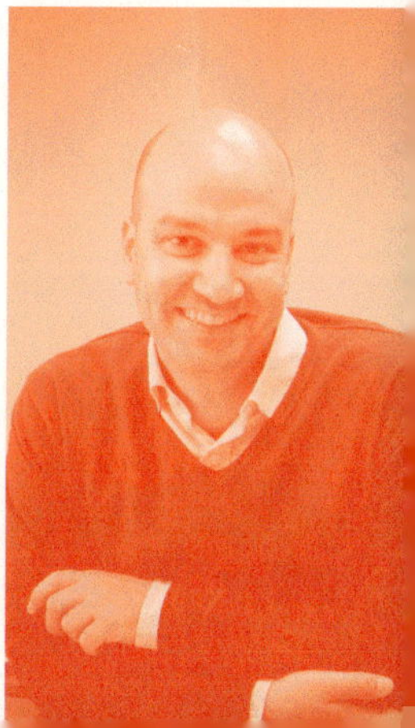

Aphasia Compendium
http://dx.doi.org/10.5772/intechopen.95198
Edited by Dragoş Cătălin Jianu and Dafin Fior Mureşanu

Contributors
Deepak Puttanna, Akshaya Swamy, Abhishek Budiguppe Panchakshari, Sathyapal Puri Goswami, Loïc Duron, Augustin Lecler, Julien Savatovsky, Raphaël Sadik, Dragoş Cătălin Jianu, Shinichiro Maeshima, Chiaki Yamaji, Rosana do Carmo Novaes-Pinto, Arnaldo Rodrigues de Lima, Silviana Nina Jianu, Traian Flavius Dan, Anca Elena Gogu, Tihomir V. Ilic, Georgiana Munteanu, Any Docu Axelerad, Claudiu Dumitru Bîrdac, Maria Kambanaros, Marina Charalambous, Hema Nagaraj, Yashashwini Channabasvegowda

First published in London, United Kingdom, 2022 by IntechOpen
IntechOpen is the global imprint of INTECHOPEN LIMITED, registered in England and Wales, registration number: 11086078, 5 Princes Gate Court, London, SW7 2QJ, United Kingdom
Printed in Croatia

British Library Cataloguing-in-Publication Data
A catalogue record for this book is available from the British Library

Additional hard and PDF copies can be obtained from orders@intechopen.com

Aphasia Compendium
Edited by Dragoş Cătălin Jianu and Dafin Fior Mureşanu
p. cm.
Print ISBN 978-1-80355-069-5
Online ISBN 978-1-80355-070-1
eBook (PDF) ISBN 978-1-80355-071-8

For EU product safety concerns:
IN TECH d.o.o., Prolaz Marije Krucifikse Kozulić 3, 51000 Rijeka, Croatia, info@intechopen.com or visit our website at intechopen.com.

Meet the editors

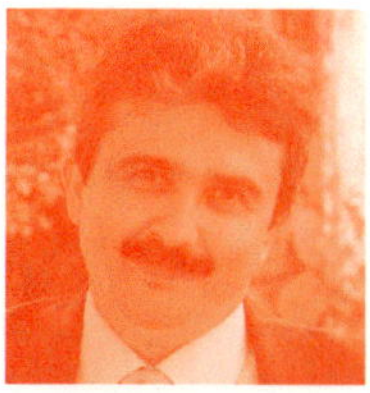

Dragoş Cătălin Jianu is a Professor of Neurology, MD, Ph.D., Dr. Habil., Ph.D. Coordinator, Head of the Centre for Cognitive Research in Neuropsychiatric Pathology, Department of Neurosciences, University of Medicine and Pharmacy, Timişoara, Romania. He has published on diverse array of topics, including vascular aphasias, vascular cognitive impairment, and neuro-ophthalmology/Color Doppler Imaging of orbital vessels (anterior ischemic optic neuropathies, central retinal artery occlusion, and giant cell arteritis with eye involvement). More recently, his work pertains to ischemic stroke: large cerebral arteries diseases/extra and transcranial Doppler sonography (TIPIC Syndrome, the carotid body paragangliomas, the congenital anomalies of the supra-aortic arteries), small cerebral arteries diseases (cerebral vessels endothelial dysfunction in patients with type 2 diabetes mellitus, and chronic kidney disease), and cerebral venous thrombosis.

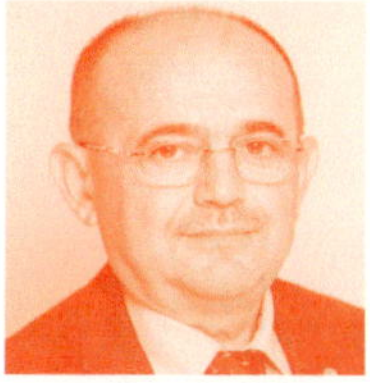

Dafin Fior Mureşanu is a Professor of Neurology, MD, Ph.D., MBA, Chairman of the Neurosciences Department, University of Medicine and Pharmacy, Cluj-Napoca, Romania, President of the European Federation of Neurorehabilitation Societies, Corresponding Member of the Romanian Academy. He has performed valuable scientific research in high interest fields such as: neurobiology of central nervous system (CNS) lesion mechanisms; neurobiology of neuroprotection and neuroregeneration of CNS; the role of Blood-brain barrier in CNS diseases; nanoparticles neurotoxicity upon CNS; cerebral vascular diseases; neurodegenerative pathology; traumatic brain injury; neurorehabilitation of the CNS; clarifying and thoroughgoing study on the classic concepts of Neurotrophicity, Neuroprotection, Neuroplasticity and Neurogenesis by bringing up the Endogenous Defense Activity concept, as a continuous nonlinear process, that integrates the four aforementioned concepts, in a biological inseparable manner.

Contents

Preface

Aphasia is an acquired central disorder of language that impairs a person's ability to understand and/or produce spoken language, often associated with impairment in reading (alexia) and writing (agraphia). Aphasia may supplementarily affect a person's ability to use musical notation, mathematical operations, and so on. Consequently, the aphasic person may present with difficulties generating and using symbol systems. Aphasia is different from a peripheral (sensory-motor) disorder of language that may mimic aphasia (such as weakness of the muscles of articulation). At the same time, it is an acquired phenomenon that appears after language has already been learned.

The most common etiology of aphasia is a stroke (80% of aphasia cases are vascular aphasias), with a prevalence of 25%–30% in acute ischemic stroke. Stroke is the third most frequent cause of death and the first cause of disability across the globe. Aphasia is considered an important marker of stroke severity, associated with a high risk of mortality, poor functional prognosis, and augmented risk of vascular dementia.

This book reviews different aspects of aphasias. It is divided into two sections including seven chapters that cover the main aspects of aphasias.

Section 1 focuses on the diagnosis of aphasias and contains four chapters.

Chapter 1, "Contributions of Linguistics to the Study of Aphasias: Focus on Discursive Approaches" by Novaes-Pinto and de Lima, discusses how aphasia disturbs not only linguistic formal levels (phonetical-phonological, syntactic, lexical-semantic) but also pragmatic and discursive aspects of language that are constitutive of meaning processes involved in the social use of language. The authors show that qualitative longitudinal research (mainly case studies) is a privileged locus to seek evidence of how linguistic levels are impacted in several forms of aphasia.

Chapter 2, "A Comprehensive Overview of Broca's Aphasia after Ischemic Stroke" by Jianu et al., discusses language and neurologic examination, diagnosis, and therapy of the patient with vascular Broca's aphasia, which is non-fluent aphasia comprising the widest range of symptoms (articulatory disturbances, paraphasias, agrammatism, evocation disorders, and discrete comprehension disorders of spoken and written language). It is considered the third most common form of acute vascular aphasia, after global and Wernicke's aphasia. Vascular Broca's aphasia is produced by infarcts or severe hypoperfusion of the superior division of the left middle cerebral artery. The reversal of hypoperfusion, following recanalization (spontaneous or secondary to thrombolysis or thrombectomy), is associated with regression of aphasia. Speech therapy is needed as soon as permitted by clinical condition. Unfortunately, pharmacotherapy remains to be evaluated. Other studies examined the potential interest of new treatments, such as transcranial magnetic stimulation.

Chapter 3, "Imaging of Vascular Aphasia" by Duron et al., reviews the state of the art of morphological and functional imaging of vascular aphasias. Magnetic resonance imaging (MRI) is the modality of choice for the etiological diagnosis of aphasia, assessment of its severity, and prediction of recovery. Diffusion-weighted imaging is used to detect, localize, and quantify the extension of the irreversibly injured brain tissue called the ischemic core. Perfusion weighted imaging (from MRI or computed tomography) is useful to assess the extension of hypoperfused but salvageable tissue called penumbra. Functional imaging (positron emission tomography, functional MRI) may help predict recovery and is useful for the understanding of language networks and individual variability.

Chapter 4, "Primary Progressive Aphasia (PPA)" by Channabasvegowda and Nagaraj, focuses on primary progressive aphasia (PPA), which is a type of dementia characterized by a loss in one or more language functions in people younger than 65 years. It is a progressive impairment of language, with the preservation of other mental processes and daily life tasks for at least two years.

Section 2 discusses outcomes and treatment of aphasias and contains three chapters.

Chapter 5, "Spontaneous Recovery and Intervention in Aphasia" by Yamaji and Maeshima, discusses the spontaneous recovery of aphasia, which occurs immediately after the onset of the disease and lasts for several months or more. The speed and degree of improvement in aphasia varies depending on the time since onset, the severity of aphasia, and each language modality. Speech and language therapy should not only promote the improvement of aphasia but also take a comprehensive approach to improving the quality of life of aphasics.

Chapter 6, "Treatment Approaches for Word Retrieval Deficits in Persons with Aphasia: Recent Advances" by Deepak et al. discusses word retrieval deficits in aphasic patients and the need for speech-language pathologists to treat this aspect of the condition. Word retrieval is an intricate process that entails various levels of processing.

Finally, Chapter 7, "The Importance of Aphasia Communication Groups" by Charalambous and Kambanaros, talks about the importance of communication buddies, who can be family members, friends, health professionals, and speech and language therapy students who serve as communication facilitators for each group member. The use of the communication buddy system, total communication approach, and systematic evaluations enables therapists to measure the effectiveness and efficacy of communication groups in terms of functional communication, social inclusion, and quality of life.

Dragoș Cătălin Jianu
Professor of Neurology, M.D., Ph.D., Dr.Habil., PhD Coordinator,
Senior Consultant Neurologist,
Department of Neurology,
"Victor Babeș" University of Medicine and Pharmacy,
Timișoara, Romania

Head of the Centre for Cognitive Research in Neuropsychiatric Pathology (NeuroPsy-Cog),
"Victor Babeș" University of Medicine and Pharmacy,
Timișoara, Romania

Head of the First Deptartment of Neurology,
Timișoara Clinical Emergency County Hospital,
Timișoara, Romania

Dafin Fior Mureșanu
Professor of Neurology, M.D., Ph.D., MBA, PhD Coordinator,
Senior Consultant Neurologist,
Chairman of the Neurosciences Department "Iuliu Hațieganu" University of Medicine and Pharmacy,
Cluj-Napoca, Romania

President of the European Federation of Neurorehabilitation Societies
Corresponding Member of the Romanian Academy

Section 1

Diagnosis of Aphasias

Chapter 1

Contributions of Linguistics to the Study of Aphasias: Focus on Discursive Approaches

Rosana do Carmo Novaes-Pinto
and Arnaldo Rodrigues de Lima

Abstract

The chapter aims to present and discuss the contributions of Linguistics to the study of aphasias, especially regarding the power of discursive theories to subsidize language assessment and therapeutic follow-up with aphasic individuals. Jakobson, in 1956, based on Saussure's approach and on Luria's neuropsychological theory, was the first scholar to call for the participation of linguists in this field, once "aphasia is a problem of language". Nonetheless, aphasia does not disturb only linguistic formal levels – phonetical-phonological, syntactic, lexical-semantic –, but also pragmatic and discursive aspects of language that are constitutive of meaning processes involved in the social use of language. Unfortunately, more traditional approaches to language assessment and to the follow-up work are exclusively based on metalinguistic tasks, which do not take into consideration the subjective and contextual aspects of language functioning. The experience we have acquired over more than thirty years within the field of Neurolinguistics has shown that qualitative longitudinal researches – mainly case studies – are a privileged locus to seek for evidences of how the linguistic levels are impacted in the several forms of aphasia. Such understanding, in turn, favor the therapeutic work towards more contextualized activities, in order to help the individuals to reorganize their linguistic-cognitive processes.

Keywords: aphasia, language, Neurolinguistics, language assessment, language therapeutic follow-up

1. Introduction

The study of aphasias by linguists started only after 1956, when Jakobson [1]—a disciple of Saussure [2]—summoned them to engage in research in the field. Also influenced by the works of Luria [3–6] in Neuropsychology, Jakobson was intrigued by the fact that scientists from different areas were interested in aphasia phenomena, while Linguistics passed over them in silence. The author blamed the linguists for "the delay in undertaking a joint into aphasia" ([1], p. 56). He was very emphatic about this issue, as we can read in the following excerpt:

> *(...) In most cases, this valid insistence on the linguist's contribution to the investigation of aphasia has been ignored. For instance, one book, dealing to a great extent with the complex and intricate problems of infantile aphasia, calls for the*

> *coordination of various disciplines and appeals for cooperation to otolaryngologists, pediatricians, audiologists, psychiatrists, and educators; but the science of language is passed over in silence, as if disorders in speech perception had nothing whatever to do with language. ([1], p. 56).*

Only a year after Jakobson's work, Noam Chomsky [7] published his famous book entitled *Syntactic Structure*, where he postulated the basis of Generative Grammar. It is important to mention that, given the context, Chomsky's theory had strongly influenced the first linguistic studies of aphasia. Indeed, most of the researches developed in the 80s settled syntax at the center of componential models and in the attempts to explain the linguistic phenomena. Agrammatism, more than any other clinical category, had gained a very special attention, once it was believed to be the result of a selective impairment of the syntactic component of language [8]. With time, investigators from other fields of Linguistics and Neuropsychology provided different explanations to agrammatism and to telegraphic speech, relating the phenomena, on the one hand, to a phonological impairment [9] or, on the other hand, as a lexical-semantic retrieval difficulty [10]. Other authors called the attention to the fact that the phenomenon is multi-componential; that is, resulting from impairments in various components and sub-components of language processing [11]. Although it has been recognized that such complex phenomena could not be approached from a single point of view, nor seen as a set of independent components, the given explanations hitherto support those theoretical models that do not account for the fact that linguistic levels are theoretical categories and, as such, are evidently of abstract nature. In other words, whether dealt within in the linguistic functioning, the linguistic levels are all intertwined and, therefore, constituents of a very complex system [12–14].

Both structuralist and generative theories, respectively postulated by Saussure and Chomsky, influenced neuropsychological models that ground most metalinguistic assessment tasks that, in turn, guide research as well as the clinical work in the field of aphasia. Thus, although such approaches may enlighten mechanisms involved in language processing, for the development of theoretical models, they do not take into consideration important aspects of language functioning – of pragmatic and discursive nature – that are relevant to shed lights on the understanding of language alterations in each concrete case of aphasia and, still more relevant, to provide adequate intervention in the rehabilitation procedures [12, 13, 15]. We will approach this topic closer, as we advance in the chapter.

On the other hand, from the 60s, a variety of currents started being developed in Linguistics aiming to account for the aspects that were downplayed by the formal theories – such as Enunciative Semantics, Pragmatics, Discourse Analysis, Conversation Analysis, among others. Such pragmatic-discursive theories turned to the individual and subjective features that take place during the social and effective use of language. Therewith, units such as "phrase", "clause" or "sentence" gave place to the concept of "utterance" [16–19].

Corollary of these new approaches to language studies, Enunciative-Discursive Neurolinguistics (henceforth: Discursive Neurolinguistics or DN) was born in the 80s at the Institute of Language Studies, due to the inaugural work of Coudry [15]. Since this is the field in which we inscribe our works, a subsection of the chapter will be dedicated to put forward, in some depth, its main theoretical-methodological principles, drawing from two data that emerged within dialogical episodes with an aphasic young woman, held at Centro de Convivência de Afásicos (henceforth: CCA) – a Center for Aphasic Individuals. Whereby, we hope to be able to explicit how pragmatic-discursive analyses come into play as an important theoretical blueprint in detecting the linguistic difficulties and alterations in each case of aphasia. Furthermore, it will have become clear how such methodology may help aphasic individuals in developing alternative processes of signification that include non-verbal utterances, especially in severe cases of non-fluent aphasias.

2. Linguistics: a brief history of the field

This section, where we will present a very brief history of the development of Linguistics, will be divided into two subsections, aiming to highlight some concepts that, somehow, run through most contemporary studies of aphasia in Neuropsychology and in Neurolinguistics.

We start subsection 2.1 pointing to a complex definition problem, which might interfere with the understanding of the main propositions of the present chapter: that is, how the word "language" should be understood along the discussion. Next, we present the main features of formal theories postulated by Saussure and by Chomsky that underlie and support, respectively, structural or componential models that have impinged on most of the studies of aphasia phenomena. Additionally to these theories, in 2.1.1, we will bring, briefly, the main contributions of Jakobson [1] to the studies of aphasia.

In 2.2, some relevant issues that ground pragmatic-discursive approaches will be addressed, driving special attention to those that subsidize our work in the field of Discursive Neurolinguistics, either in research, as well as in the language follow-up with aphasic individuals.

2.1 Formal theories and the establishment of models

When Saussure inaugurated the so-called "scientific study of language", in the beginning of the twentieth century, he distinguished 'langue' from 'langage'. By the first term, present in several Latin languages (in Portuguese: *língua*, Italian: *lingua*, Spanish: *lengua*), he meant "the structure of a particular idiom". Whereas, the conception of 'langage' (in Portuguese: *linguagem*, Italian: *linguaggio*, Spanish: *lenguaje*, is broader than the first, referring to a very complex human activity, "heteroclite and multifaceted", being at the same time physical, physiological, psychological [2]. According to Saussure, the study of language, as a human activity, demands knowledge from different areas, such as Psychology and Anthropology among others [20].

In a saussurean stance, the *langue* is understood as one of the manifestations of the *langage*, and conceived of as a system of signs: a set of units that are related to each other within a whole. Besides this distinction, another dichotomy posed by the author is 'langue' *versus* 'parole' – the latter meaning 'speech' –, related to the individual usage of the 'langue', including its motor activity, dialect variations, among other features. So, the 'langage' would be constituted by 'langue' + 'speech'. The scientific project of Saussure defined the study of the 'language system' (the 'langue' itself) as the scope of Linguistics, having the objectivity as the central epistemological aspect. In the words of the author: "Whereas speech is heterogeneous, *the langue*, as defined, is homogeneous. It is a system of signs in which the only essential thing is the union of meanings and sound-images, and in which both parts of the sign are psychological" ([2], p. 15). Throughout the chapter, the distinctions between 'langue' and 'langage' will be recalled, when necessary.

Most of the linguistic approaches born later in the twentieth century disagreed with the distinctions posed by Saussure – mainly concerning the dissociation between *langue* and *parole*. Nevertheless, such programmatic ideas hitherto persist and abound, for instance, in didactic school materials and also in clinical contexts – grounding the formulation of language assessment tests, as well as of therapeutic manuals, privileging isolated units as "words" and "phrases". We will turn to this issue, in more detail, while presenting the core concepts of Discursive Neurolinguistics – in Section 3.

Another formal theory that has strongly impacted neuropsychological works regarding language functioning was inaugurated in 1954 by Chomsky [7], and is known as Generative Grammar. The approach spawned a new dichotomy in Linguistics – 'competence', by one hand, and 'performance', on the other. Whereby, the scientist defined 'competence' as the innate and implicit set of mental knowledge that a speaker of any natural language has at his/her disposal; that is, a species-specific capacity. From a set of limited grammar rules, the speaker generates an infinite number of grammatical sentences and is able to recognize those that would be agrammatical. This theoretical principle works also as a methodological tool for Neuropsychology and Neurolinguistics, and derive, for instance, the grammaticality judgment tests so well known in the studies of agrammatism and telegraphic speech [12].

The concept of 'performance', in its turn, would correspond to the linguistic behavior that results not only from the implicit knowledge of the language, but also from extra-linguistic factors, such as social conventions, beliefs, emotional attitudes from the speaker, assumptions about the interlocutor's attitudes, besides psychological and physiological processes involved in language production [20].

Despite not been formulated with the specific aim of grounding studies on language acquisition nor on language pathologies, very quickly Chomsky's theory started being applied to these fields, exploring the concepts of 'competence' and 'performance', as well the distinction between the 'principles' and the 'parameters'. The 'principles' are universal and would correspond to the innate set of grammar rules that a speaker has, independently of his language (the 'langue'), while the 'parameters' would be the features (syntactic and lexical-semantic) acquired along the experience of the individual with a specific language.

Due to the belief in the independence and primacy of syntax, Chomsky's followers started postulating a great number of models aiming to lay bare how the different subcomponents of syntax operate and/or interact, in order to produce grammatical sentences. The Generative Grammar is a very strong theory in contemporary Linguistics and also guides a substantial amount of works in Neurolinguistics, which are interested in the various linguistic-cognitive processes, such as lexical retrieval, agrammatism, word-finding-difficulties, and the like [13]. Many of such syndromes or symptoms are approached considering they are either the result(s) of an impaired component, which would disturb the linguistic 'competence' [8, 11] or as the consequences of adaptation processes when the individuals need to face their linguistic difficulties. Language models in Generative Theory are computational, and, therefore, also exclude its social and contextualized use.

In the next subsection, we will present – even if briefly – the contributions of Jakobson [1] to the studies of aphasia. The author is also placed in Section 2, not only because we are considering the strong influence of Saussure's structuralism on his theory, but especially because he established the linkage between the language system and its functions [21]. In other words, he started a functionalist approach to language, which he applied to the study of aphasia; and, furthermore, that we also articulate in our methodological procedures of analysis.

2.1.1 Jakobson: contributions for the studies of aphasia

> *If aphasia is a language disturbance, as the term itself suggests, then any description and classification of aphasic syndromes must begin with the question of what aspects of language are impaired in the various species of such a disorder. This problem, which was approached long ago by Hughlings Jackson (1915), cannot be*

> *solved without the participation of professional linguists familiar with the patterning and functioning of language ([1], p. 3).*

Jakobson's approach to language may be conceived of as a functionalist structuralism and, therefore, it is also somehow limited for explaining the complex discursive nature of language, as we will point later in this chapter. The author aimed to explain the "two aspects of language" that, when impacted, generate the "two (main) types of aphasia" [1]. His approach to aphasia was strongly influenced by the Lurian Neuropsychology, author that also grounds our work in Neurolinguistics. We highlight Jakobson's project of applying linguistic theory to aphasia problems, citing his own words:

> *Speech implies a selection of certain linguistic entities and their combination into linguistic units of a higher degree of complexity. At the lexical level this is readily apparent: the speaker selects words and combines them into sentences according to the syntactic system of the language he is using; sentences in their tum are combined into utterances ([1], p. 5).*

Based on the two different operations postulated by Saussure [2]: 'selection' and 'combination', Jakobson sought to explain the main difficulties present in two opposite types of aphasia: *agrammatism* and *jargonaphasia*.

Agrammatism, on one hand, is produced due to an impairment of the operation of combining linguistic units into the syntagmatic/metonymic axis of language, generating, for instance, the telegraphic speech. Jargonaphasia, on the other hand, results from difficulties related to the selection of a specific unit from a set of other possible concurrent possibilities, in the paradigmatic/metaphoric axis of language, deriving, for example, the production of a paraphasia: the substitution of a target word by another, semantically or phonologically related. Jakobson points out that the majority of real cases could be placed between the two extreme ends of the axes, once the axes are projected over each other during the production of an utterance. In such a way, the author, indeed, criticized Saussure for his belief in the linear nature of language production [1].

It is relevant to point that Jakobson expanded many of Saussure's principles and dichotomies. It is worth mentioning that he made explicit the relationship between the system and the context of its production, contributing to develop the previous existing models of the so-called "Information Theories", which postulated the roles of "the "speaker", of the "receiver", of the "code" and of the "channel" in the schemes that represented the interaction between two participants. Jakobson highlighted that, besides being used to denote and name objects and their relations (the *referencial* function), language also has the role to communicate something to someone – a message, a feeling, or even a thought – (the *communicative* function), to establish and/or maintain a social contact (the *phatic* function), to show social position, to manipulate a situation or someone, to convince people, and the like (*connotative* or *appellative* function). The emphasis also can be cast on the speaker (emissary) himself, to his motivation to speak (*emotive* or *expressive* function). The other functions postulated by Jakobson were the *poetic* – when the focus is the on the message itself, on its different possibilities of saying something and, finally, the *metalinguistic* function, when the emphasis is on the linguistic code [21, 22].

The latter, which is specially explored for the elaboration of language assessment tests and for therapeutic follow-up manuals, is, therefore, only one of the linguistic functions, which refers to the possibility to pinpoint a specific part of the discourse – a word or a grammar feature – to describe it, and to explain it. It is, in other words, the use of language to talk about itself. Although the metalinguistic aspect is relevant and constitutive of language functioning, it should by no means be conceived of as the representative of the underlying complexity of linguistic-cognitive functioning [15, 23].

Another concept developed by Jakobson, regarding aphasia phenomena, is the one of "translation", which has been mobilized by Discursive Neurolinguistics and concerns the fact that aphasic individuals frequently recur to non-verbal signs (body expressions, drawings or deictic gestures) in order to refer to the verbal signs that they cannot select and/or combine while trying to produce meaning within interactional and dialogical processes [24].

Despite some criticisms made to Jakobson's structural view of interactions, as beforementioned, we argue that the author needs to be recognized for his enormous contributions to the understanding of the functions of language – which would be lately developed by other linguistic approaches, such as the Discursive Functionalism [25] – and, evidently, for proposing a linguistic explanation to aphasia and to its semiology.

In the next subsections we will present and discuss some theoretical-methodological principles to which we recur in order to argue in favor of a discursive approach to aphasia and, also, to ground our criticisms towards most language assessment and follow-up tasks with individuals in this pathological condition.

2.2 Discursive approaches: focus on the social use of language

As we have seen in the previous section, for formal theoreticians Linguistics should focus their studies on the 'langue', on the system itself, as postulated by Saussure, or as a mental knowledge of grammar rules – the competence of the speakers –, as posed by Chomsky, leaving aside any extra-linguistic factor to describe it and explain it.

Possenti [14], when criticizing the structuralism, stated that such project cannot be achieved once that, even seen from its interior, language (the langue) is not a plain surface, a perfect object, whose functioning "could be calculated independently from the factors that would affect it from outside, in determined conditions" ([14], p. 20). Languages are not internally uniform; they vary in practically all domains (phonology, morphology, syntax and lexicon). Despite the recognition of such levels according to specific laws, they cannot be conceived of as independent and, in a certain way, not completely different from each other. In the words of the author:

> *A phonological change may affect the morphological level immediately; the attribution of one or another meaning to a word may implicate in a different syntactic organization; the simplification of a verbal inflectional system may, for instance, produce a syntactic change (obligatory subject role). This means that the fact of a problem being typically dealt with within one level does not imply that only such a level results affected ([14], p. 21).*

Furthermore, languages as systems are opaque. The interpretation of linguistic units will always depend on a certain amount of implicit and redundancies that are present in concrete utterances. There is no guarantee of a controlled and unmistakable interpretation of any linguistic production. On the contrary, "interpretations are the result of a complex calculation of linguistic and pragmatic-discursive factors" ([14], p. 20).

For Bakhtin [18, 19] – another critic of Saussure's structuralism – even if one takes words as isolated units we must consider that they are, in general, polyphonic. The real unit of communication, for the author, is the 'utterance' that emerges only in dialogical contexts. This issue will be more explored in the next section, when we approach the field of DN.

As for Pragmatics, its inaugural work is considered the publication of the first edition of the Journal of Pragmatics, in 1977, by Haberland & Mey [26]. The authors define the field as the study of the concrete use of language, with emphasis on the linguistic practices by its users. Pragmatics is the Science of Language Use [27, 28], and, therefore, broadens the interests of Linguistics to the 'langage', rather than restricting it to the 'langue'.

Thus, Pragmatics seeks to lay bare the relationship between the structure of a specific language and its use, within the context of social production [28]. Concepts of 'society' and of communication', backgrounded by formal models, gained special attention, and non-conventional elements were included in the explanation of linguistic facts [27, 28].

Among the most important researchers in the field, Austin has to be underlined, for his theory of the Speech Acts that, in brief, relates what is said to what is done – that is, what we say by doing and what we do by saying. Language is understood as an activity constructed by the interlocutors. It is impossible to discuss language without considering the act of language itself, the act of speaking. Language is not the description of the world, but the action itself [29]. Pragmatics is a field that holds a great diversity of interests and has sheltered authors such as Benveniste [16], and Grice [30], spawning the inauguration of other fields, such as Argumentative Semantics and Conversation Analysis. It is worth mentioning that Peirce [31], author who is most known for his works in Semiotics, was the first to use the word "Pragmatics", in 1878, in his work "How to make our ideas clear". The author explored the relationship between the signal and its reference (object) and also related the sign to his interpretant – that is, to whom the sign means. Later, in 1969, it was the work of Searle [32], in Speech Acts, that mostly influenced Linguistics.

Of all the principles pointed by Searle, we underline that of "cooperation" that guides the interaction and which is very relevant for the establishment of meaning in dialogical episodes with aphasic individuals, as we will point out in our data analysis.

At this point, it is relevant to make clear that when we state that our approaches are oriented by discursive theories, we refer to this wide range of works that include Enunciative Semantics, Discourse Analysis, Conversation Analysis and Pragmatics. All of them have in common the fact that the linguistic analysis cannot refer to the language as an independent structure, free of the participation of speakers and their very specific contexts of production.

Needless to say that Linguistics, as a scientific field, has been very fruitful, especially because of interdisciplinary interests, among them Neurolinguistics. The aim of bringing some of the concepts and main theories to this chapter was, as previously mentioned, to highlight the contributions of Linguistics to different approaches to aphasia, either for researchers who work with processing models and explore formal language theories or to those who conceive of language as an activity in which the subjects have the main role of 'work' on the linguist resources to produce meanings [17, 18, 33].

3. Discursive neurolinguistics

As it has been already made explicit in the beginning of the chapter, Coudry [15] criticizes the fact that many researchers try to understand language in aphasia by looking through the slit of formal theories, what considerably reduces its complexity. The direct application of what the author calls the "frozen knowledge of linguistic concepts" by Neurolinguistics and Neuropsychology fulfills the psychometric demands of those fields [34]. The focus of such approaches is put on isolated words and sentences evaluated strictly by means of metalinguistic tasks –, which, in its turn, influence the semiology, the diagnosis and also the therapeutic follow-up in pathological conditions. As models, they are acceptable and may give indices of how some aspects of language have been impaired due to a brain lesion, but they cannot be directly related to the language complexity in its social and concrete use. As Bakhtin argued, if someone attempts to use a model to represent the "whole" of language functioning, such enterprise would be "science fiction" [18, 23, 35].

Coudry provided an inventory of metalinguistic tasks that usually compound the language assessment batteries, which involve isolated linguistic units as phonemes, words, sentences, letters, syllables, and the like; as we can see in the following summary: repetition of phonemes or monosyllabic words (after the investigator or from a printed list); repetition of logatomes (non-words in the language, but which follow its phonological pattern); spelling and repetition of words; discrimination between minimal pairs; forming words from initial phonemes; naming objects orally or by written form; identifying an object among others in pictures; making lists following a particular order (months of the year, days of the week, etc); checking verbal fluency (through lists of names; animals, flowers or any other category within the time lapse of one minute); defining words given by the examiner; describing a picture; understanding simple or compound sentences; explaining proverbs; reading aloud (words, sentences or paragraphs); copying words or sentences; writing under dictation; etc. [15, 35].

According to Coudry "the success or failure of the aphasic subject in one or more of the aforementioned tests serve as criteria to classify the individuals into a type of aphasia" ([15], p. 9). Despite the statistical correlations established by empirical studies, the author emphasizes that, for certain purposes, the tests could serve to the typological diagnosis, but "only for the diagnosis". A symptom or a group of symptoms allows a classification but does not explain the underlying processes of a phenomenon and, even more important, does not provide clues for the reorganization of language, as meaningful and contextualized activities [15, 35]. These claims are bounded up with a dynamic concept of language. Franchi [33], a linguist who influenced in a very important way the Neurolinguistics developed at IEL, described language as a 'constitutive activity'. It does not only constitute the individuals, but also the language system (the langue) itself. Subjects continuously "work" on the language material resources (phonemes, words, morphemes, grammar rules) to produce their discourses (concrete utterances), within a determined social-historical-cultural background [17, 18, 33].

Still on linguistic-cognitive assessment, it is noteworthy to point that, based on the results of psychometric tests, aphasic individuals are classified also into broader categories, such as "fluent" or "non-fluent". A classic example is the famous "Cookies Theft picture" [36]: a description task in which the subject is supposed to describe the scene given in a card, within the time lapse of one minute. The score is established by the number of words produced by the individual, irrespective of whether the utterances are or not understandable and/or comprehended by an interlocutor. Such methodological approaches have been of concern to DN and been criticized since the inaugural work of Coudry [12, 13, 25, 33, 35, 37]. As for the (non-)fluency classification to aphasia, we have claimed that, as argued by Scarpa [38, 39], fluency is a myth; an abstract concept, usually compared to the written and finished form of a text or to the production of an "ideal subject". Hesitations, word finding difficulties, and TOT phenomena, for example, are present also in the speech of non-aphasic individuals, to different degrees, and are always related to pragmatic aspects – such as the speech genre, the asymmetric conditions established during an interaction, the motivation to speak, the knowledge of the participants about the discursive topic, the shared knowledge between the interactants, and so on [38–42].

It has yet to be stressed that Discursive Neurolinguistics, since its inauguration, sets out to explain the phenomena by addressing inter-subjectivity as a primordial aspect in the constitution of linguistic-cognitive functioning. In this respect, Mazuchelli [43] clarifies that since the majority of studies still assume an epistemological dissociation of brain, body, and subjectivity, one of the most challenging theoretic-methodological aspects of this approach is to address the complexity of a non-idealized subject.

Therefore, the investigations go beyond its constitutive sciences – Neurosciences and Linguistics – and articulate interdisciplinary assumptions held by different scientific fields, such as Psychology, Anthropology, Philosophy, Philosophy of Language, Semiotics, Public and Community Health, Demography, Sociology, among others [44]. It goes without saying that there is much more to set out about the theoretic-methodological assumptions of our socio-historic-cultural perspective. However, since space limitations precludes a detailed discussion of all these features, before rounding off this topic, we would like to address just one more central aspect of our approach to aphasia – the relevance of qualitative methodology.

In the beginning of the 80's, when settling the principles for Discursive Neurolinguistics, Coudry stated that only longitudinal and qualitative approaches, which take into consideration the aspects that are preserved in the language system, as well as the subject's pragmatic and discursive competence, are adequate to cast light on the complexity of aphasia phenomena [15, 35, 45].

Contrary to what it may seem, "qualitative analyses demand rigorous control and frequent verification; it consists of a continuous process in order to look for cases to contradict findings as well as evidence to support them (...)". "Results are not simply interesting observations; they are carefully verified cumulative outcomes negotiated across multiple sources and perspectives" ([46], p. 685). A last feature of qualitative approaches to be highlighted is that research "unfolds as data are collected and analyzed resulting in a cyclical and flexible process". In such approach, "the investigator collects, analyzes and verifies data, identifies phenomena of interest, then continues to collect and analyze data to progressively narrow the investigation and hone in on phenomena of interest" (...) and, thus, "seeks to discover whatever emerges as important to the understanding of the phenomenon under study" ([46], pp. 682–683). Our data and analysis, in the next section, aim to illustrate closely these issues brought by the authors and so far emphasized in this chapter.

4. CCA: a center of interaction for aphasic individuals

We start this section defining the locus of our work with aphasic individuals and presenting some principles that ground its foundation. Afterwards, we will bring data of two dialogical episodes with an aphasic individual – referred by means of the acronym GB.

CCA is fruit of a partnership established in 1989 between the Institute of Languages Studies (IEL) and the Medical Sciences Faculty (FCM) at the University of Campinas, São Paulo, Brazil, aiming to help individuals to surpass the conditions imposed to them by aphasia. It is a center for interaction among aphasic and non-aphasic subjects: researchers, caretakers, families, therapists, under-graduate and post-graduate students. It is an institutional alternative to integrate aphasics in their social groups [15]. Indeed, the acronym CCA stands for "Centro de Convivência de Afásicos", being "convivência" a word that does not have an exact correspondence in English, and that means "to live with" or "co-living".

There are three CCA groups at the moment, under the supervision of the professors who respond for the field of Neurolinguistics, in the Department of Linguistics. Each group is very heterogeneous regarding the individuals that participate of the activities, their types of aphasia and the degrees of severity. It is important to mention that the subjects are not classified into a clinical category, neither according to etiological causes, nor to oral or written production/understanding impairments. In our approach, heterogeneity is constitutive of human relations and is, in fact, what mostly enriches our interactions [35].

Concerning the reorganization of language, the individuals are encouraged to talk about themselves, and about a great diversity of quotidian themes (routines, life in family, national and/or international news, soccer or other sports, politics, and the like). The activities usually involve the use of different speech genres (narratives – autobiographic, fables, jokes –, argumentation, poetry, proverbs, letters, journalistic language, charges, among others). "By doing so, at the same time they expose their linguistic-cognitive difficulties – as everyone has a turn to express an opinion, bringing up something to share – they are oriented/helped in order to (re) organize language, memory, attention" ([35], p. 237).

Conversation is the social situation in which people do most of their talking [47]. The absence of conversational success is a primary determiner of negative social stigma and handicap. Qualitative approaches "have highlighted the importance of collaboration within the conversational interactions of dyads that include an individual with aphasia and an individual without aphasia ([47], p. 668)". Conversation is a collaborative operation carried out by two or more participants; it is social and collaborative in character. During a conversation, utterances are produced in response to – or in relation to – a prior one, organized in a turn-by-turn sequential basis, which is not a mechanical structure. The interlocutors within the dyads overcome problems that emerge along a conversation in a cooperative way, and the aphasics are encouraged to proceed to self-repair, which makes it evident that they preserve a communicative competence.

All the sessions of CCA individual or in the group meetings are video-recorded and the utterances are afterwards transcribed (discursively and/or phonetically, depending on the type of aphasia and the specific needs of each research) or described, when the meaning is made up of non-verbal strategies. The data are analyzed having the microgenetic paradigm as a parameter. Besides being a methodology to help the individuals (re)organize their linguistic-cognitive abilities, the analysis lead to the discursive theorization about aphasia [35].

Aiming to illustrate our theoretic-methodological approach, we bring two episodes of the same aphasic individual — GB – from two different moments of her participation at CCA: (i) when she attended the meeting for the first time, in 2016 [25] and (ii) more recently, during an online meeting, held in 2021 [48]. After presenting both data, we will proceed to the analysis and to our final considerations.

Needless to say that the episodes are rather long, due to the discursive perspective of 'building meanings in cooperative processes', in a dyad of an aphasic individual and a non-aphasic one. We argue that episodes 1 and 2 (**Tables 1** and **2**) are comparable, not only because they refer to the production of the same aphasic individual (GB), but also because they verse about the same topic – the day that GB had the Cerebral Vascular Accident (henceforth: CVA), which was reported to different interlocutors, after a lapse of time of more than four years. During all this period (from 2016 to 2021), GB has been participating of individual and group sessions of CCA, where the linguistic processes impaired by aphasia were substantially reorganized. It is worth mentioning that stories about the neurological episode have been described in literature as highly reportable [49], as we also have noticed in many of our CCA participants.

i. GELEP database - [GB_23/08/2016:_Narrating the neurological episode at the first interview] – time lapse: 04′27″

Turn	Interlocutor	Utterances by GB and Imp	Comments
01	**Imp**	**Tell us a bit about yourself, GB. What did happen to you?**	
02	GB	*No, uh: car: no, look! [GB shows three fingers in her hand] three:: seat down [makes gesture indicating distance with her hand] far away. #Refife>	# Recife, capital of Pernambuco, Brazil.,
03	Imp	<Recife!, that's right Wow! Did you go by car?	*
04	GB	Yep!	
05	Imp	That's why you showed here [point to the word "Recife" written on a sheet of paper] for me, right? Recife is in?	
06	GB	Pernambuco No, look! [GB wrote the word "#Ceará" on a sheet of paper]	# Ceará is a brazilian state
07	Imp	Ceará? Who is from Ceará?	
08	GB	Father.	
09	Imp	Your father?	
10	GB	Yep! *Drove; later:: >	
11	Imp	< First, you went to Ceará! >	
12	GB	<Yep! Me too:: >	
13	Imp	< Wow, you too! Did you share? Your father and you driving?	
14	GB	Yep	
15	Imp	Right; Ceará And, from Ceará you went to /re...	
16	GB	*fife*>	Recife
17	Imp	<Recife! So, you were traveling a lot!	
18	GB	Oh:: Yep!	
19	Imp	And then, you got in Recife:: >	
20	GB	< *Beach:: sea:: [writes down the word "Saturday" on the sheet of paper], right!?	
21	Imp	Ok, Saturday?	
22	GB	Yep! *Morning [writes down the word "morning" on the sheet of paper] morning:: *eated... [points towards herself with her finger]	* Mistaken form of the verb.
23	Imp	<You?	
24	GB	Yep.	
25	Imp	So, woke up early: ate. And then?	
26	GB	*"Mother, look:: to sleep" [make gesture as if she was sleeping by laying her head on her hand]" "- It's nice": right?	
27	Imp	Woke up too early: so went back to bed.	
28	GB	[makes a gesture as if she were drawing a board on air] tevilision* [writes down the word "TV" on the sheet of paper] "-Please!" [she makes gesture as if she was pressing the buttons of the remote] >	*for television

i. GELEP database - [GB_23/08/2016:_Narrating the neurological episode at the first interview] – time lapse: 04′27″

Turn	Interlocutor	Utterances by GB and Imp	Comments
29	Imp	< turn on?	
30	GB	Yep! [gestured as if she were trying to hold something] *Mouth, nope! [pointed towards herself with] *Speech [pointed towards herself] nope! [head shaking]	
31	Imp	Suddenly!?	
32	GB	Suddenly!	
33	Imp	Didn't you feel anything?	
34	GB	*Hey, look:: head, pain!	
35	Imp	I see, so you had a headache?	
36	GB	Yep:: Fat!	
37	Imp	Were you overweight?	
38	GB	Yep.	
39	Imp	But, the headache, were you in pain since the day before?	
40	GB	Yep. Ouch, a lot!!	
41	Imp	So, it was really painful?	
42	GB	Yep.	
43	Imp	So, you "woke up" normally, had breakfast >	
44	GB	<Yep	
45	Imp	And then, when you tried to turn on the TV you could no longer move yourself. And then, really fast, you went to the hospital?	
46	GB	Yep	
47	Imp	How about when you got there?	
48	GB	*Ouch! Questions: no, look: mother!	
49	Imp	Ok, they asked to your mother And, did they suspect that you were having a CVA, when you got there?	CVA: Cerebral Vascular Accident
50	GB	No!	
51	Imp	Didn't they?::	
52	GB	No!	
53	Imp	But, were you waiting?	
54	GB	*Later:: another:: hospital	
55	Imp	Ok, changed the hospital and went to another one?	
56	GB	Yep GP!	GP: General Practitioner Center.
57	Imp	All of it, on Saturday?	
58	GB	Yep.	
59	Imp	First, you came over to GP and later to a hospital?	
60	GB	Yep.	
61	Imp	But, at the hospital, did they figure out that you had had a CVA?	

i. GELEP database - [GB_23/08/2016:_Narrating the neurological episode at the first interview] – time lapse: 04′27"

Turn	Interlocutor	Utterances by GB and Imp	Comments
62	GB	No, look! [gestured "something slow" with her hand]	
63	Imp	But, did you get hospitalized soon?	
64	GB	Ouch! yep!	
65	Imp	But, was it right on Saturday?	
66	GB	Yep.	
67	Imp	So, you mean that they examined you and then reached the conclusion that you'd had a CVA	
68	GB	Yep [pointed towards her exam results and, later, towards her head].	
69	Imp	Did they do tomography? Was it tomography, wasn't it?	
70	GB	Yep.	
71	Imp	When you arrived at this hospital, did they immediately give any medication to you?	
72	GB	Yep:: on a drip, right?	
73	Imp	Which medication?	
74	GB	Do not know	
75	Imp	That's ok.	

Notes about the transcriptions:
The signs ">" and "<" correspond to the moments when one utterance overlaps, interrupts or crosses the other person's production.
The symbol ":" means there was a short pause, while "::" means a longer pause.
The symbol "" stands for agrammatical utterances or for paraphasias produced by GB.*
The symbol "#" refers to places in Brazil, identified in the comments.
Descriptions given in brackets correspond to GB's non-verbal utterances.
The acronyms "Imp" and "Iar" stand for the non-aphasic interlocutors, whereas GB is the acronym for the aphasic individual.

Table 1.
Episode 1: dialogical process between Imp and GB.

The transcription given above of a conversation with GB, first of all, allows us to notice the predominance of telegraphic style utterances, considering that, in most of her turns, they consist of a single word or by the combination of a few content words from open classes: nouns, adjectives, verbs, whereas they lack functional words from closed classes (prepositions, articles, conjunctions, connectors) and also bound morphemes, such as noun and verbal inflections.

GB's utterances are mainly produced to agree or disagree with the interlocutor Imp. For instance, she answers using only the word "yep" in 21 utterances from the total of the 36 turns: 04, 10, 12, 14, 18, 22, 24, 30, 36, 38, 42, 44, 46, 56, 58, 60, 64, 66, 68, 70 and 72. She uses the single-word "nope" in utterances 50 and 52. In all of them, she agrees with the information given by Imp. In some of these utterances, however, she expands the answers with telegraphic style utterances, like in turns: 10, 12, 22, 30, 36, 56, 68 and 72. Sometimes the expansion is done with a gesture or by writing a word related to the answer that she wants to give, such as in 02, 06, 22, 26, 30, 68 and 69. Sometimes GB answers with a monolexematic word or by saying very short utterances: 08 (father.), 10 (drove: later::), 12 (mee too::), 17 (Recife!), 20 (*beach:: sea::), 26 (mother, "look:: to sleep" it's nice"::, right?), 36 (fat!), 56 (GP) and 72 (on a drip, right?). It is interesting to notice that in turns 28 and 68, for instance, GB's answers are produced almost exclusively with gestures, which we also consider as utterances, grounded by Bakhtinian theories.

It is relevant to mention that Imp, a speech therapist from CCA, had already been told a lot about GB's neurological accident from the anamneses carried out with GB's mother, two weeks before the session in which episode 1 took place. That is the reason why Imp is the one who provides most of the information concerning the narrative: *when* it happened, *how* it happened, *where* she was, *who* was with her, *which* were the symptoms, *what* they have done to help her, and so on.

Although GB's utterances are mostly monolexematic, as already pointed, she was very cooperative and contributed substantially to the process of meaning construction, producing telegraphic speech or recurring to face expressions and deictic gestures.

Recurring to Jakobson's explanation of aphasia, we notice she had either a problem to select words to express her speech will, as well as difficulties to combine them into a grammatical utterance. GB, while in the group sessions, often used to say that she was aware that another word would come into the place of the one she wanted to utter. Such situations made her feel ashamed to speak. We oriented her to say whatever word that would come, even it was not the desired one, because in this way we also could have a hint about her *speech will* and could help her in the process of building signification. As Luria has pointed, paraphasias produced by aphasic individuals are usually produced by semantic or by phonological ties.

After presenting the second episode, we will proceed to the comparative analysis of both narratives and, right after, will bring our final considerations concerning the contribution of a discursive approach of language to the understanding of aphasias.

i. GELEP database - [GB_12/05/2021:_Narrating the neurological episode to Iar]
Time lapse: 06'53"

Turn	Interlocutor	Utterances by GB and Iar	Comments
01	Iar	[...] can you tell me what happened on the day you had the CVA? Because I do not know this story. What happened?	
02	GB	Yep... see. I traveled:: >	
03	Iar	< And	
04	GB	*Traveled. Then, three days, car. Right?	
05	Iar	Where did you traveled by car?	
06	GB	# Matão to #Ceará.	Matão, the district where GB lives. Ceará, a Brazilian state
07	Iar	You went from Matão to Ceará?	
08	GB	Ceará, Tauá >	Tauá, an inner in Ceará.
09	Iar	< Tauá?	
10	GB	Tauá, three days. So, I: ate too much:: You know? *Sleeping.	
11	Iar	Eating and sleeping!	
12	GB	Yep:: Then, Ceará, Tauá: Stayed twenty days:: Huum, I do not know. *Then, my aunt. Mother sister. "Let us go Recife?" It's quite close, is not it? Kind of close, right? Eleven hours!	Mother's sister
13	Iar	So, did you travel from Ceará to Recife?	
14	GB	Yep!	

i. GELEP database - [GB_12/05/2021:_Narrating the neurological episode to Iar]
Time lapse: 06'53"

Turn	Interlocutor	Utterances by GB and Iar	Comments
15	Iar	Who was driving?	
16	GB	Father.	
17	Iar	And...	
18	GB	It's because:: I: drive too. But:: very dangerous, you know?	
19	Iar	Ok, got it. Then, did you all go to Recife?	
20	GB	Yep. *Then, Monday, arrived Recife:: Then, Saturday, ten o'clock:: Before: nine o'clock. Recife, Saturday, happened the CVA.	
21	Iar	So, you all arrived on a Monday and spent a week >	
22	GB	< Yep! >	
23	Iar	< So, in the weekend, on Saturday, that you had the stroke?	
24	GB	Yep!	
25	Iar	But, were you already feeling unwell?	
26	GB	*Much pain, pain in: in: *Dipirona* no! Much:: Oh my Gosh:: Pain, you know? Pain, pain. Strong pain, indeed! >	Dipirona is a painkiller
27	Iar	< Where was such a pain?	
28	GB	Head, you know?	
29	Iar	Ok, you got a strong headache. But was it on the day or you had been in pain days before?	
30	GB	Before. Three days: *"Mom, see, strong headache", you know?	
31	Iar	Yep, got it!	
32	GB	Then, Dipirona! I was also stubborn, right?	
33	Iar	Stubborn? Why stubborn?	
34	GB	Well, because:: drugstore, you see? (they) told GP, you see?	
35	Iar	But did not you check your blood pressure, nor anything else in those days?	
36	GB	Nope! Dipirona only!	
37	Iar	So, what did happen on Saturday? What did you feel specifically?	
38	GB	*Well, arm, TV: Then, the zapper, held it:: How can I say? Flipped through the shows, you know?	
39	Iar	Did you switch the channel?	
40	GB	*Yes! Then, hand weak, you see? Leg weak. Then, voice I no longer had. Then, my mother held me.	
41	Iar	So, this was the moment you realized that you were feeling unwell?	
42	GB	Really unwell! And, detail: *Aunt Mary, you do not know her. Apartment! >	
43	Iar	< Apartment? >	
44	GB	< Apartment, high!	
45	Iar	Ouch! How did you get downstairs? In the elevator?	
46	GB	No! on the stairs! Cousin held me: mom also held me, you see? Ouch, a real hassle!	

i. GELEP database - [GB_12/05/2021:_Narrating the neurological episode to Iar] **Time lapse: 06'53"**			
Turn	**Interlocutor**	**Utterances by GB and Iar**	**Comments**
47	Iar	I can imagine! Luckily, it's now behind you, phew!	
48	GB	*Then, cousin: GP: After hospital	
49	Iar	So, did you go to the GP and later to the hospital?	
50	GB	Yep!, then it took too long, you know?	
51	Iar	Phew, luckily everything got fine!	
52	GB	Indeed! I'm speaking, it's good!	

Table 2.
Episode 2: dialogical process between Iar and GB.

Despite the fact that Iar – a linguist, non-aphasic interlocutor – was acquainted with the narrative produced by GB in 2016 [25], the topic was brought up again as a methodological tool, seeking to understand how GB had organized her linguistic processes after being a participant of CCA. Many activities were developed with GB aiming to help her to expand her utterances. In our point-of-view, the language reorganization is evident in the analysis of her utterances. In the second episode, only in a few of them she answers "yep", as in turns 02, 14, 22, 24, 31, 40, 46 and 50 and "nope" in turns 36 and 46. However, they are followed, in almost all of them, by additional and new information, even if by means of monolexematic utterances.

Despite the presence of some agrammatic utterances, as in turns 4 (*Traveled. Then, three days, car. Right?), 10 (So, I ate too much:: You know? Sleeping.), 12 (Then, my aunt. Mother sister. "Let's go Recife? It's quite close, isn't it?" Kind of close, right?), 20 (Then Monday arrived Recife:: Then, Saturday, ten o'clock:: Before: Nine o'clock. Recife, Saturday, happened the CVA). Similar processes take place in turns 26, 30, 34, 38, 40, 42, 46, 48 and 50.

Some linguistic elements that were completely absent in the first episode, such as prepositions, in the second episode came up, as in turns 4 and 6, as well as the accurate finite forms of the verbs, in turns 2 and 4 (traveled), 10 (ate, sleeping), 20 (arrived), 34 (told), 38 and 40 (held), 50 (took) and 52 (speaking). There also connectors, as in turns 20 and 40 (then), as well as in turn 52 (and).

Differently from the first episode, in this dialogical process, GB is the more informative interlocutor, insofar as Iar helps her to organize the events in her narrative. We highlight, in the table below (**Table 3**), some of the following telegraphic style utterances, where GB constructs her narrative exploring the 'word order' of the content words, revealing a great improvement in the processes of selecting and combining the linguistic elements. In other words, we can claim that GB became a much more competent narrator.

02	Yep... see. I traveled:: >
04	*Traveled. Then, three days, car. Right?
06	# Matão to #Ceará.
08	Ceará, Tauá >
10	Tauá, three days. So, I: ate too much:: You know? *Sleeping.
12	Yep:: Then, Ceará, Tauá: Stayed twenty days:: Huum, I do not know. *Then, my aunt. Mother sister. "Let us go Recife?" It's quite close, is not it? Kind of close, right? Eleven hours!
18	It's because:: I: drive too. But:: very dangerous, you know?

DOI: http://dx.doi.org/10.5772/intechopen.101058

20	Yep. *Then, Monday, arrived Recife:: Then, Saturday, ten o'clock:: Before: nine o'clock. Recife, Saturday, happened the CVA.
26	*Much pain, pain in: in: Dipirona no! Much:: Oh my Gosh:: Pain, you know? Pain, pain. Strong pain, indeed! >
30	Before. Three days: *"Mom, see, strong headache", you know?
32	Then, Dipirona! I was also stubborn, right?
38	*Well, arm, TV: Then, the zapper, held it:: How can I say? Flipped through the shows, you know?
40	*Yes! Then, hand weak, you see? Leg weak. Then, voice I no longer had. Then, my mother held me.
42	Really unwell! And, detail: *Aunt Mary, you do not know her. Apartment! >
46	No! on the stairs! Cousin held me: mom also held me, you see? Ouch, a real hassle!
48	*Then, cousin: GP: After hospital
50	Yep!, then it took too long, you know?
52	Indeed! I'm speaking, it's good!

Table 3.
Telegraphic style utterances taken from Episode 2.

The dialogical work in dyads, as we have been arguing, allows the aphasic individual to achieve his/her speech will or, in some cases, to get closer to it. The qualitative approach, as already pointed, demands a rigorous analysis of data in order to investigate the phenomena of interest. The microgenetic analysis grounded on the postulations of Vygotsky [50, 51] allowed us, concerning the two episodes above, to pinpoint the elements that reveal the processes that underlie GB's difficulties and also the alternative resources she articulates (verbal and non-verbal) in order to achieve her speech will. Aiming to understand the dynamics of a process, Vygotsky argued that it is necessary to find the 'genesis' of a given phenomenon and observe its development. The paradigm is known as "microgenetic" because it is oriented to "indicial details" and not referring to the short duration of the events. It is 'genetic' in the sense of being historical, by focusing on the movements that take place during processes and because it seeks to relate singular events with other plans of culture, social practices, circulating discourses, institutional spaces, etc. [52].

Bounded up with our discursive musings, such a paradigm is the most appropriate one to account for data that come up in interactions among socio-cultural and historically situated individuals. Concerning aphasia, it is evident that the etiology and the local of the lesion should be considered in the genesis of the linguistic processes and impairments. However, together with organic features, there are socio-cultural aspects that constitute the individuals, usually disregarded by traditional approaches [35].

5. Final words

Observing aphasia in real interaction episodes is like seeing a movie in slow motion, as it allows us to uncover aspects of language functioning that could not be detected and recognized in normal speech and in its complex dynamics. Coudry's work aimed, at first, to confront hegemonic aphasiology and speech therapy, especially regarding the methodology of language assessment and therapeutic follow-up [15], as we have tried to show along the chapter.

We agree with Possenti [14], when the author states that the relashionship between two interdisciplinary fields is often problematic and, certainly, asymmetric. A sociolinguist, for instance, presumably studies more Linguistics than

Sociology, while a sociologist probably does the opposite. About the field of Neurolinguistics, Possenti [14] raises the following question: Would it be possible for a neurolinguist to have a balanced comprehension of Neurology and also of Linguistics? He does not believe so; neither do we. To begin with, each field is substantially complex and, furthermore, our interest is more turned to one or to the other field. According to the author, this fact does not mean, however, that it would be impossible to postulate relevant problems in each field, even within asymmetric specializations. The author emphasizes that the phenomena are too complex to be approached from a single point of view. No theory or model would account for all its relevant aspects, as we have discussed.

Aphasiological tradition and Neurolinguistics restricted their efforts to assess language in aphasia to some aspects of metalinguistic knowledge, which influenced the semiology, the diagnosis and also the treatment of language pathologies.

Explanations for most neuropsychological language disturbs have been limited to how brain episodes impact the linguistic levels (phonological, syntactic and lexical-semantic), although Hughlings Jackson [53], in the beginning of the twentieth century, and Luria [5] had already detected pragmatic and discursive aspects of such alterations. At that time, such problems had been noticed and related to 'problems of thinking', once Linguistics would be restricted to the scope of the language system – the langue [54].

We would like to end this chapter mentioning that the latest works sheltered by the Group of Studies of Language in Aging and in Pathologies (GELEP), to which we belong, have contributed to the understanding of clinical categories [12, 25, 35, 37, 44, 48] and other phenomena in aphasia, from which we underline the tip-of-the-tongue (TOT) [55], the production of paraphasias [56] and paralexias [57], the analysis of language in aging, along with the discussions of linguistic prejudice against communities with vulnerabilities [43].

Ethical issues, along all those theoretical-methodological questions presented and discussed along the text, have a very central role in our research in Discursive Neurolinguistics and in our extension works at CCA. For this reason, we end this chapter citing the valuable words of Lyon:

> *Treatment should not be a process of a person, but of people. It should not be a process of just language and communication repair, but of facilitating purpose and meaning in life and strengthening ties with others in those natural life contexts that matter the most ([58], p. 689).*

Acknowledgements

We are very thankful to Coordenação de Aperfeiçoamento de Pessoal de Nível Superior (CAPES), the Grants Agency that funded the publication charges for this chapter. Still in an institutional level, our thanks go to Fundação de Amparo à Pesquisa do Estado de São Paulo (FAPESP) for furthering our research by means of the following grants: 2017/26777-2 and 2019/24150-8 and to Conselho Nacional de Desenvolvimento Científico e Tecnológico (CNPq), by means of the grant number 311920/2017-9. Special thanks are addressed to Isabella Tardin Cardoso, coordinator of the Post-Graduation Program in Linguistics; who, for extension, stands for on behalf of the whole staff of the Institute of Language Studies (IEL), University of Campinas.

DOI: http://dx.doi.org/10.5772/intechopen.101058

Author details

Rosana do Carmo Novaes-Pinto* and Arnaldo Rodrigues de Lima
Department of Linguistics, University of Campinas, São Paulo, Brazil

*Address all correspondence to: ronovaes@terra.com.br

References

[1] Jakobson R. Two aspects of language and two types of aphasic disturbances. In: Jakobson R, Halle M, editors. Fundamentals of language. Gravenhage: Mouton & Co; 1956. p. 55-76.

[2] Saussure F. Curso de Linguística Geral [Course in General Linguistics]. São Paulo: Cultrix; 2004. 279 p.

[3] Luria A. The working brain. London: Penguin Books; 1973. 398 p.

[4] Luria A. Cognitive Development: its cultural and social foundations. Massachusets: Harvard University Press; 1976. 272 p.

[5] Luria A. Basic Problems of Neurolinguistics. The Hague: The Gruyter Mouton; 1976. 407 p.

[6] Luria A. Pensamento e Linguagem: as últimas conferências de Luria [Thought and Language: the last conferences of Luria]. Porto Alegre: Artes Médicas Ed; 1986. 251 p.

[7] Chomsky N. Syntactic Structures. The Hague: Mouton; 1957. 117 p.

[8] Grodzinsky Y. The syntactic characterization of agrammatism. Cognition. 1985; 16: 99-120.

[9] Kean M L. Agrammatism: a phonological deficit? Cognition. 1979; 7: 69-83.

[10] Goodglass H, Menn L. Is agrammatism a unitary phenomenon? In: Kean, M L. Agrammatism. New York: Academic Press; 1985. p. 1-26.

[11] Caramazza A, Berndt R. A multi-component deficit view of Agrammatic Broca's aphasia. In: Kean, M L. Agrammatism. New York: Academic Press; 1985. p. 898-918.

[12] Novaes-Pinto R. Contributions from the discursive study to the critical analysis of clinical categories [thesis]. Campinas, SP: University of Campinas; 1999.

[13] Novaes-Pinto R. Do fonológico ao discursivo: hipóteses sobre a produção da chamada 'fala telegráfica'no contexto das aphasias [From phonological to discursive: hypothesis on the production of the so-called 'telegraphic speech'in the context of aphasias]. Estudos Linguísticos. 2020; 49: p. 135-151. DOI: 10.21165/el.v49i1.2624.

[14] Possenti S. Língua: sistema de sistemas [Language: a system of systems]. In: Damasceno B, Coudry M I, editors. Temas em Neuropsicologia e Neurolinguística [Themes in Neuropsychology and Neurolinguistics]. São Paulo: TecArt; 1995. p. 20-25.

[15] Coudry, M I. Diário de Narciso: discurso e afasia [The Diary of Narciso: discourse and aphasia. São Paulo: Martins Fontes; 1988. 284 p.

[16] Benveniste E. Problemas de Linguística Geral [Problems in General Linguistics]. Campinas: Pontes Ed; 1988. 387 p.

[17] Voloshinov V. Marxism and the Philosophy of Language. Austin: University of Texas Press; 1986. 224 p.

[18] Bakhtin M. Speech Genres & Other Late Essays. Austin: University of Texas; 1979. 177 p.

[19] Bakhtin M. Toward a Philosophy of the Act. Austin: University of Texas; 1972. 132 p.

[20] Petter M. Linguagem, língua, linguística [título em inglês?]. In: Introdução à Linguística Teórica: objetos teóricos. São Paulo: Contexto; 2002. p. 11-24.

[21] Jakobson R. Linguística e Poética [Linguistics and Poetics]. In: Jakobson R. Linguística e Comunicação [Linguistics and Communication]. São Paulo: Cultrix; 2007. p. 118-147.

[22] Barros D. A comunicação humana [The human communication]. In: Fiorin L. Introdução à Linguística: objetos teóricos [Introduction to Linguistics: theorethical objects]. São Paulo: Contexto; 2002. p. 25-54.

[23] Novaes-Pinto R. Desafios metodológicos da pesquisa em Neurolinguística no início do século XX [Methodological challenges in neurolinguistic research in the beginning of the twenty-first century]. Estudos Linguísticos. 2011; 40: 966-980.

[24] Coudry M I. Neurolinguística Discursiva: afasia como tradução [Discursive Neurolinguistics: Aphasia as translation]. Estudos da lingua(gem). 2008; 6: 7-36.

[25] Lima, A R. As palavras funcionais na chamada fala telegráfica em enunciados de sujeitos afásicos [thesis]. Campinas, S.P: University of Campinas; 2017.

[26] Haberland H, Mey J. Editorial: linguistics and pragmatics. Journal of Pragmatics. 1977; 1: 1-12.

[27] Pinto J. Pramática [Pragmatics]. In: Mussalin F, Bentes A, editors. Introdução à Linguística: domínios e fronteiras [Introduction to Linguistics: domains and borders]. São Paulo: Cortez; 2001; 2: p. 47-68.

[28] Fiorin L. A linguagem em uso [Language in Use]. In: Fiorin L. Introdução à Linguística: objetos teóricos [Introduction to Linguistics: theorethical objects]. São Paulo: Contexto; 2002. p. 165-186.

[29] Austin J. How to Do Things with Words. Oxford: Oxford Paperbacks; 1962. 178p.

[30] Grice P. Studies in the way of words. Cambridge: Harvard University Press; 1989. 398p.

[31] Peirce C. Prolegomena to an apology for pragmaticism. In: Piece C. The of Interdisciplinarity. City: The monist; 1906. p. 492-546.

[32] Searle J. Indirect speech acts. In: Syntax and Semantics. New York: Academic Press; 1975. p. 59-82.

[33] Franchi C. Linguagem – Atividade Constitutiva [Language – Constitutive Activity]. Cadernos de Estudos Linguísticos. 1992; 22: 09-39. DOI: 10.20396/cel.v22i0.8636893.

[34] Coudry M I. Neurolinguística e Linguística [Neurolinguistics and Linguistics] In: Temas em Neuropsicologia e Neurolinguística [Themes in Neuropsychology and Neurolinguistics]. São Paulo: TecArt; 1995. p. 12-19.

[35] Novaes-Pinto R. A social-cultural approach to aphasia: Contributions from the Work Developed at a Center for Aphasic Subjects. In: Unner T, editor. Latest findings in Intellectual and Developmental Disabilities approach. Riejka: InTech; 2012. p. 219-244. DOI: 10.5772/28256.

[36] Goodglass H, Kaplan E. Boston diagnostic aphasia examination booklet. Philadelphia: Lea & Febiger; 1983.

[37] Lima A, Novaes-Pinto, R. A chamada "fala telegráfica" e sua relação com as dificuldades de encontrar palavras: uma reflexão a partir de enunciados de sujeitos afásicos não-fluentes [The so-called "telegraphic Speech and its relation with the word finding difficulties: a reflection from the utterances of two non-fluent aphasic subjects]. Estudos Linguísticos. 2017; 46: 715-729. DOI: doi.org/10.21165/el.v46i2.1624.

[38] Scarpa E. Sobre o sujeito fluente [On the fluent subject]. Cadernos de Estudos Linguísticos. 1995; 29:163-180.

[39] Scarpa, E. (Ainda) sobre o sujeito fluente [(Still) on the fluente subject]. In: Lier de Vitto M F, Arantes L, editors. Aquisição, Patologias e Clínica da Linguagem [Acquisition, Pathologies and Clinic of Language]. São Paulo: EDUC; 1995;1: 161-180.

[40] Scarpa E, Novaes-Pinto R. Contribuições para o estudo da (dis) fluência [Contributions to the study of (dis)fluence]. Cadernos de Estudos Linguísticos. 2012; 54: p. 5-9.

[41] Novaes-Pinto R. O conceito de "fluência" nos estudos das afasias [The concept of "fluency" in the studies of aphasia]. Cadernos de Estudos Linguísticos. 2012; 54: 117-134. DOI 10.20396/cel.v54i1.8636975.

[42] Novaes-Pinto R, Santana A P. Semiology of aphasias: A critical discussion. Psicologia: Reflexão e Crítica. 2009; 22 (3): 413-421. DOI 0.1590/S0102-79722009000300012.

[43] Mazuchelli L P. Stereotypes and representations: discourses on and in ag(e)ing [thesis] Campinas, S.P: University of Campinas; 2019.

[44] Lima A R. Enunciados de estilo telegráfico nas afasias: funcionamento linguístico-cognitivo sob uma visão integrada dos níveis linguísticos [Telegraphic style utterances in aphasia: linguistic-cognitive functioning under a linguistic levels integrated view]. Estudos Linguísticos. 2020; 49: 860-882. DOI 10.21165/el.v49i2.2628

[45] Novaes-Pinto R. Qualitative Research in Neurolinguistics: the case of Word Finding Difficulties and related phenomena. Cadernos de Estudos Linguísticos. 2018; 60: 425-451. DOI: 10.20396/cel.v60i2.8653310.

[46] Simmons-Mackie N, Damico J S. Qualitative methods in aphasia research. Aphasiology. 1999; 13: 681-687. DOI 10.1080/026870399401786.

[47] Damico J, Oelschlaeger M, Simmons-Mackie N, Qualitative methods in aphasia research: conversation analysis. Aphasiology. 1999; 13: 667-679. DOI: 10.1080/026870399401777.

[48] Lima A R. Estudo neurolinguístico da produção de enunciados de estilo telegráfico nas afasias: o desafio de compreender as variações inter- e intracasos. [A neurolinguistic study on telegraphic style utterances in aphasia: the challenge of understanding inter- and intra-case variations]. [thesis]. Campinas, S.P: University of Campinas; (forthcoming).

[49] Ochs E, Capps L. Living narrative: Creating lives in everyday storytelling. Massachussets: Harvard University Press; 2001.

[50] Vygotsky L. A formação social da mente [The History of the Development of Higher Mental Functions]. São Paulo: Martins Fontes; 1991. Xx p.

[51] Vygotsky L. Pensamento e Linguagem [Thought and Language]. São Paulo: Martins Fontes; 1987. Xx p.

[52] Góes M C. A abordagem microgenética na matriz histórico-cultural: uma perspectiva para o estudo da constituição da subjetividade [The microgenetic approach in the historical-social matrix: a perspective for the study of the constitution of subjectivity]. Cadernos Cedes. 2000. v. 50, p. 9-25.

[53] Jackson H. On affections of Speech from Disease of the Brain. In: Jackson H. Papers on affections of speech. Brain. 1879. p. 203-222.

[54] Damasceno B. Neuropsicologia da atividade discursivo-pragmática em

sujeitos com lesões frontais [Neuropsychology of the discursive-pragmatic activity in subjects with frontal lesions]. In: Temas em Neuropsicologia e Neurolinguística [Themes in Neuropsychology and Neurolinguistics]. São Paulo: TecArt; 1995. p. 1-11.

[55] Oliveira M V B. The tip-of-the-tongue phenomenon: a neurolinguistic approach [thesis]. Campinas, SP: University of Campinas; 2015.

[56] Souza-Cruz, T C. Em briga de marido e mulher ninguém mete... o garfo: a neurolinguistic study of the production of semantic paraphasia in aphasic subjects [thesis]. Campinas, SP: University of Campinas; 2013.

[57] Boccato D M A. Paralexia: understanding the phenomenon through a case study in the context of aphasias [thesis]. Campinas, SP: University of Campinas; 2018.

[58] Lyon J. A commentary on qualitative research in afasia. Aphasiology. 1999, p. 681-687.

Chapter 2

A Comprehensive Overview of Broca's Aphasia after Ischemic Stroke

Dragoş Cătălin Jianu, Tihomir V. Ilic, Silviana Nina Jianu, Any Docu Axelerad, Claudiu Dumitru Bîrdac, Traian Flavius Dan, Anca Elena Gogu and Georgiana Munteanu

Abstract

Aphasia denotes an acquired central disorder of language, which alters patient's ability of understanding and/or producing spoken and written language. The main cause of aphasia is represented by ischemic stroke. The language disturbances are frequently combined into aphasic syndromes, contained in different vascular syndromes, which may suffer evolution/involution in the acute stage of ischemic stroke. The main determining factor of the vascular aphasia's form is the infarct location. Broca's aphasia is a non-fluent aphasia, comprising a wide range of symptoms (articulatory disturbances, paraphasias, agrammatism, anomia, and discrete comprehension disorders of spoken and written language) and is considered the third most common form of acute vascular aphasia, after global and Wernicke's aphasia. It is caused by a lesion situated in the dominant cerebral hemisphere (the left one in right-handed persons), in those cortical regions vascularized by the superior division of the left middle cerebral artery (Broca's area, the rolandic operculum, the insular cortex, subjacent white matter, centrum semiovale, the caudate nucleus head, the putamen, and the periventricular areas). The role of this chapter is to present the most important acquirements in the field of language and neurologic examination, diagnosis, and therapy of the patient with Broca's aphasia secondary to ischemic stroke.

Keywords: language, aphasia, Broca's aphasia, ischemic stroke, vascular aphasia

1. Introduction

Aphasia that acquired central disorder of language, which alters the patient's capacity of understanding and/or producing spoken and written language, occurs in about one-third of the patients with acute stroke (ischemic or hemorrhagic). The language disturbances are frequently combined into aphasic syndromes, contained in different vascular syndromes. Still, aphasia subtype is changeable and may undergo variations over time: in the acute stage of the recovery, the most common type of aphasia is the global one; during the first year after stroke, anomic aphasia seems to be the most common aphasia subtype. In fact, anomia denotes the most important aphasia manifestation and long-term vascular aphasia consequence [1].

Broca's aphasia (after Goodglass-Kaplan classification), known also as "motor cortical aphasia" (Lichtheim), "efferent or kinetic motor aphasia" (Luria), "expressive aphasia" (Déjerine, Albert, Pick, Weissenburg, McBride), "phonematic aphasia" (Hécaen), "Broca aphasia—the common form" (Lecours & Lhermitte), "verbal aphasia" (Head), "syntactic aphasia" (Wepman & Jones) is a non-fluent aphasia, comprising the widest range of symptoms: articulatory disturbances, paraphasias, agrammatism, evocation disorders, and discrete comprehension disorders of spoken and written language. It is a type of aphasia whose primary, trademark feature is considered to be the disability of spelling words (word evocation disorder), leading thus to impaired fluency and agrammatism (deficit in formulating and processing syntax) [2, 3]. Several studies concluded that in acute first-ever stroke, the frequency of Broca's aphasia is from 10 to 15%, being the third most frequent type of aphasia after global aphasia (almost 30%) and Wernicke's aphasia (almost 16%) [2, 4–6].

2. Clinical aspects

The different levels of the language (phonetic, phonemic, morphemic, morpho-syntactic, semantic, and pragmatic) can be differentially affected in the various types of language disturbances. For instance, Broca's aphasia is significantly associated with grammatical defects (so-called agrammatism in Broca's aphasia), whereas the semantics of nouns is impaired in posterior fluent aphasias [3].

The different aphasia subtypes are characterized by specific language disturbances. In the evaluation of each patient who presents with aphasic language disorders, the following aspects must be followed: the assessment of oral output/spontaneous speech, the assessment of repetition, the assessment of comprehension, and last but not least, the assessment of reading (lexia) and writing (graphia).

2.1 Language assessment

2.1.1 Assessment of oral production (spontaneous speech)

2.1.1.1 Fluency

In the absence of aphasic mutism or when mutism has regressed, the patient presents a non-fluent, unwieldy verbal output, characterized by difficulties to initiate spontaneous speech, effortful, with hesitations and slow output (10–15 words/min), and interrupted by frequent word-finding pauses. Sometimes, he presents dysprosody, remarking a monotonously oral expression, with the absence of melodic modulation [2, 5–11].

2.1.1.2 Presence of deviations at various levels

a. Sound/arthric level (incorrect articulation of a sound)—dysarthria.

- Patients with Broca's aphasia are having difficulties in precisely making articulatory movements, resulting in a lot of phonetic abnormalities (incorrect production of phonemes), occasionally ensuing the so-called "foreign accent" or "pseudo accent" [2, 3].

b. Phonemic level (omission, addition, substitution, inversion of a phoneme)—phonemic paraphasias.

- Phonological paraphasias are the result of the apraxia of speech [3];
- even thought it could be argued that apraxia of speech is not exactly a language defect [3].

c. Verbal level (naming):

- Semantic (verbal) paraphasias;
- Word-finding difficulty (anomia), especially in spontaneous speech;
- Deficits in action naming being more severe than deficits in object naming.

d. Syntactic level:

- Agrammatism (frequently more obvious afterward the acute phase): oversight of functional/grammatical words (conjunctions, articles, prepositions, auxiliary verbs/e.g., "the," "an," and inflections), while conceptual words (verbs, adverbs, and nouns) are used more frequently, resulting in the so-called "telegraphic speech." From time to time, the oral output can be limited to a few stereotypical terms (e.g., "tan tan") [2, 8, 11–13].

2.1.2 Assessment of repetition

In patients with Broca's aphasia, the humble repetition is characteristic. The repetition of operational words and flexional endings is difficult, resulting in phonemic and verbal paraphasias (e.g., "My mother reads a book"/"mother-read-book"). Repetition and naming are impaired, although this is less marked than spontaneous speech.

Automatic speech consisting of numbering from 1 to 10, enumerating the days of the week, the months of the year, repeating a poem, can spectacularly ameliorate the verbal fluence [11, 14, 15].

2.1.3 Assessment of oral comprehension

Comprehension is preserved in most Broca aphasic patients. Good oral comprehension (the patient easily manages to perform the examiner's tasks/commands) allows the complete evaluation of language components. In some cases, syntactic comprehension can be more difficult, especially when the examiner requests for understanding more complex sentences or to perform multiple commands [6]:

a. Distinguishing between different operational words ("in," "on," "under," "over") is almost impossible.

b. Comprehension of passive reversible sentences can be affected [12, 16].

Examples:
(Q): "The girl was kissed by the boy. Who kissed whom?
(A): Girl kiss boy."
(Q): "The chicken was eaten by the dog. Who ate whom?
(A): Chicken eat dog."

2.1.4 Assessment of reading and writing

Reading and writing are furthermore compromised [14]. Receptive lexia is more affected than oral comprehension. Frontal alexia—literal alexia, was first described by Benson [8] and represents the incapacity in recognizing and naming individual letters, though full words are well recognized. In some cases, a deep central alexia is noticed, with incapacity of reading nonexistent words [17]. Lexia of abstract words or operational words is more difficult than that of concrete or conceptual words [17].

Regarding the graphia, it is also impaired in patients with Broca's aphasia. It is not only the result of right hemiplegia, as long as it is also present in patients without motor deficit. Graphia shows changes similar to those of the oral expression, but with different intensity. There are troubles of writing spontaneous or dictated texts, while the copied graphia is relatively well conserved. Agraphy has central (linguistic) and peripheral elements [11]. Discaligraphy, literal and/or grapheme paragraphs are observed; there is a tendency toward agrammatism of variable intensity (thus operational words and inflectional endings are omitted) [18]. After a while, dissociation between a reduced oral language, with agrammatism, and jargon-agraphia phenomena occurs, causing a succession of incomprehensible paragraphias [19].

In conclusion, there are three determinant characteristics representing the essence of Broca's aphasia: preserved comprehension, agrammatism, and dysarthria [2, 5–8].

2.2 Associated signs and symptoms

2.2.1 Contralateral hemiparesis (right hemiparesis/hemiplegia)

Lesions that cause Broca's aphasia also interrupt adjacent cortical motor fibers and deep fiber tracts, this type of aphasia being usually associated with a motor defect in the right hemi body. The hemiparesis [20]:

- affects especially the hand and the face, the leg being less affected;
- moreover, it is more distal than proximal (affecting the hand muscles more than the shoulder ones);
- being caused by a lesion situated at the level of the upper motor neuron, in most cases, the hemiparesis is characterized by an increased muscle tone (spastic hemiparesis);
- its severity is variable, depending on the extension of the cerebral lesion;
- may have impact over the articulatory organs (lips, tongue, cheeks), usually leading to a spastic dysarthria (upper motor neuron injury). This type of dysarthria is characterized by imprecise consonants, monotonous tone, reduced stress, rough voice, mono loudness, and a sluggish speech rate.

2.2.2 Apraxia of speech

Apraxia of speech represents a deficiency in planning and programming the sequences of movements necessary in speech production. Along with agrammatism, it is considered as another essential clinical element in the diagnosis of Broca's aphasia.

It is characterized by abnormalities in phoneme production (phonetic deviations), omissions, and substitutions of speech sounds, leading to decreased speech rate (non-fluent speech, evoked with difficulty). Automatic language (counting from 1 to 10, counting the days of the week, the months of the year) is preserved; instead, repetition is clumsy [20]:

It can be associated with bucco-facial apraxia (difficulties in planning and performing facial and mouth movements on request: to open the mouth, to blow air, to move the tongue) and/or dysarthria.

The patient is aware of his problem, unsuccessfully trying to correct his disturbance by effort. Instead, he presents difficulty in initiating statements, awkwardness articulatory movements. The patient is presenting articulatory variation, repeating attempts of the same expression.

2.2.3 Frontal acalculia

Patients with prefrontal injuries frequently develop calculation difficulties that are not easily detected. Patients with damage in the prefrontal areas of the brain may display serious difficulties in mental operations, successive operations (particularly backward operations; e.g., 100–7), and solving multistep numerical problems. Written arithmetic operations are notoriously easier than mental operations. Difficulties in calculation tasks in these patients correspond to different types [20]:

- Attention difficulties

    i. are reflected in the patient's difficulty in maintaining concentration on the issue;

    ii. result in defects in maintaining the conditions of the tasks and impulsiveness in answers;

- Perseveration

    i. is observed in the tendency to continue presenting the very same response to different conditions;

    ii. can be found in extrasylvian (transcortical) motor (dysexecutive) aphasia;

- Deficiency of complex mathematical concepts.

2.2.4 Depression

The patient with Broca's aphasia is aware of his oral expression disorder, developing feelings of helplessness and frustration, with a slightly irascible frame of mind, eventually leading to anxiety and depression [5–7], adding much more struggle in the recovery process of language.

3. Anatomo-clinical correlations

Broca's aphasias are generally the consequence of infarcts (usually embolic) in the anterior superficial sylvian territory of the dominant hemisphere for language. Other causes are cranio-cerebral trauma, cerebral hemorrhage, and less frequently, multiple brain metastases or infiltrative multiform glioblastomas. In the last two conditions, the spontaneous evolution is toward global aphasia.

Lesions or dysfunctions usually involve the left side of the brain in right-handed individuals [21], precisely the following structures:

a. Broca's area:

- the posterior part of the third frontal gyrus (F3)—Brodmann areas 44 and 45.
- lesions in this area determine transitory apraxia of speech.
- larger lesions, involving besides Broca's area the subjacent white matter, produce transient mutism, quickly followed by an improving syndrome with noticeable arthric distortions and difficulties in action naming rather than in object naming.

b. Rolandic operculum:

- inferior part of the motor area: Fa.

c. Lesions can extend or individually affect:

- the insular cortex and subjacent white matter;
- centrum semiovale;
- capsulostriatum (head of caudate nucleus and putamen);
- periventricular areas.

Ischemic lesions comprising together these structures and Broca's area can produce the complete syndrome of Broca's aphasia. Broca's aphasia is produced by infarcts/severe hypoperfusion of the superior division of the left middle cerebral artery (MCA) (**Figures 1** and **2**) [2, 5, 6, 22–24].

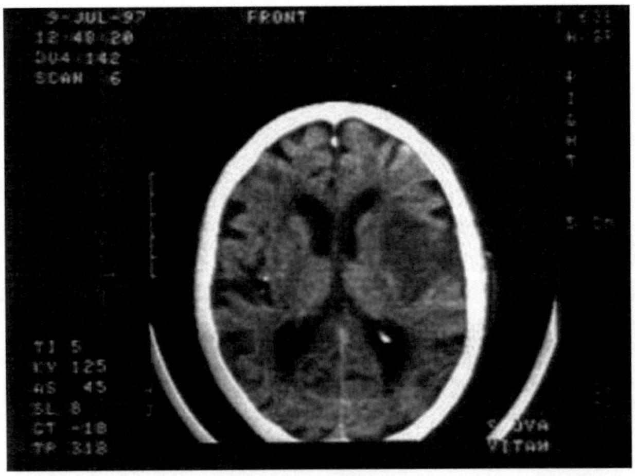

Figure 1.
Example of native brain CT scan of a Broca aphasic patient, showing a hypodense area of 3.5/3 cm arranged in the left frontal region, affecting the frontal operculum (operculum frontale), the frontoparietal one (operculum fronto-parietale), the island, a portion of the underlying white matter and the putamen [2].

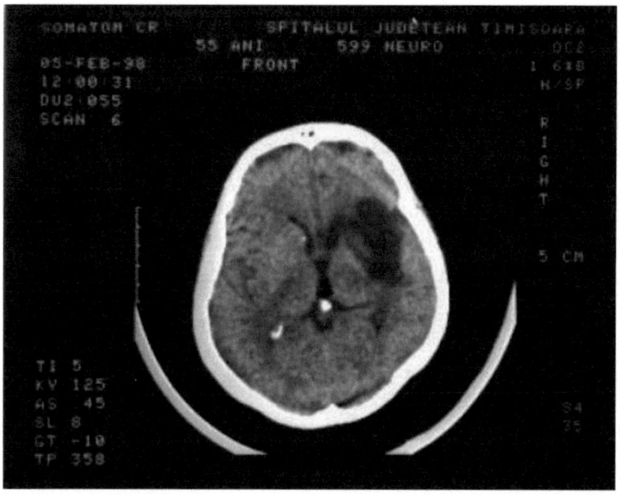

Figure 2.
Example of native brain CT scan of a Broca's aphasic patient, revealing a hypodense area of 5/4 cm with left frontal location [2].

During the last two decades, there were conducted different studies that were meant to study the hypothesis that during the acute period of the stroke, the lesion's location is the main conclusive factor in establishing the type of aphasia. Kreisler et al. pointed out in their study that imaging supported the classical anatomic localization (for example: lesions situated in the left inferior frontal gyrus might lead to Broca's aphasia and lesion situated in the left superior temporal gyrus might lead to Wernicke's aphasia). Furthermore, their study concluded that non-fluent aphasia was correlated with lesions of postero-inferior frontal gyrus, the putamen, centrum semiovale, and the inferior parietal lobule; repetition disorders were associated with injuries of external capsule and posterior internal capsule, and difficulty in finding words was related with injuries of anterior and posterior language areas or with the subcortical structures [25]. There are other studies conducted by Godefroy et al. and Z.-H. Yang et al., which also pointed out that the most significant factor in establishing the aphasia type was the lesion's site [26, 27].

On the other hand, there are some studies that found out that a great number of aphasia types were not concordant with the classical neuroanatomical site of expression and comprehension [28, 29].

Concluding, there are two hypotheses [30]:

- One that sustains that the language center is the liable core for language (though, the brain mechanism of language functions is not restricted to that limited area of the cerebral cortex);

- Another one that sustains that wide-ranging areas related to language are the connection of the language functions and that coordination and close interconnection between these two components have made it possible for people to carry out complex and various language activities, so necessary for human communication.

Language system of the brain is a wide, complex network, and this topic requires further investigation.

Different imaging techniques have been used to precisely specify the site of the brain lesion responsible for aphasic syndromes: diffusion MRI (diffusion tensorimaging—DTI: tractography—used in detecting the course of a specific nerve fiber bundles), MRI diffusion-weighted imaging (especially helpful in detecting the areas of acute infarction, soon after the clinical stroke onset—within 15–20 min), functional MRI (fMRI—quantifies hemodynamic changes associated with active metabolism during ongoing neuronal activity; as the linguistic areas are activated, more oxygen is consumed in those areas, resulting in release of greater amounts of deoxyhemoglobin), positron emission CT (PET—detects radioisotopes injected into the bloodstream and reaching to specific areas of the brain). However, there are still needed complex studies to establish this multifaceted language process [31].

4. Evolution of Broca's aphasia

Primarily, the patient is unable to release any sound (mutism), with a tremendously impaired comprehension (global aphasia) or, in opposition, almost normal. In evolution, stereotypes can sometimes be installed, which consist of the involuntary repetition of a syllable, a word, or even a phrase, in the absence of any other expression [6, 8, 18, 19, 32–34].

In rare situations, the regression of language disturbances stops at the level of monotonous permanent stereotypes (without prosody) and without semantic significance. In some old Broca aphasias, stereotypes with semantic significance, with hyperprosody and, possibly, with rich gestures can be observed. In most cases, however, the evolution is favorable, the patient developing the typical clinical picture of Broca aphasia [18, 32]. Subsequently, there is a partial restoration of verbal fluency (hereinafter, slow fluency), with decreased articulation disorders and those of evocation of conceptual words (lexical enrichment) [2]. Voluntary-automatic dissociation occurs and the language begins to convert into propositional [2]. Sometimes, the evolution is toward agrammatism, other times toward motor transcortical aphasia or motor amnestic aphasia [19].

Studies have reported better recovery in Broca's and conduction aphasia, lower rates of recovery in global and anomic aphasia [4, 35, 36]. A study completed by Mazzoni et al. supported the idea that comprehension has a better recovery than expression [37], whereas Basso et al. reported that transcortical sensory aphasia had a worse prognosis than Broca's or transcortical motor aphasia [38]. El Hachioui et al. related that different levels of the language improve at different times, as phonology recovers earlier than semantic or syntactic language, and comprehensive language recovers earlier than expressive language [39].

5. Therapeutical approach in Broca's aphasia

5.1 Pharmacological therapy

At the moment, in acute ischemic stroke, the rapid reestablishment of cortical perfusion (i.v. thrombolysis/endovascular therapy—thrombectomy) during the first 4.5 h (thrombolysis), and 6–12 h (thrombectomy) from the clinical onset, represents the most efficient acute treatment approach. Several large randomized clinical trials have shown significant value in outcome with intravenous thrombolysis [40] or endovascular therapy [41]. Although all these studies were not designed to specifically assess the language's evolution, a secondary investigation of a large randomized clinical trial of endovascular therapy (Multicenter Randomized Clinical Trial of Endovascular Treatment for Acute Ischemic Stroke in the Netherlands; MR CLEAN) [42] has proven that the language score on NIHS

Scale gained points (0–2 points) in the intervention group, compared with the control group. Hillis et al. conducted a small randomized clinical trial, which demonstrated that temporary rise of blood flow early after left hemisphere stroke due to large vessel occlusion or severe stenosis was related to language improvement [43].

In chronic post-stroke Broca's aphasia, no other pharmaceutical intervention has proven its efficacy, since no randomized study has been able to demonstrate their efficiency [44]. Nevertheless, there are some trials that showed that there are some medications that have improved the results of speech therapy. The main idea of these studies is that recovery of language depends on neuroplasticity, which might be stimulated by administrating medications that modulate neurotransmitters [45]. Studies have proven that behavioral interventions can lead to neural reorganization. Even more, this process is facilitated by some neurotransmitters such as: acetylcholine, dopamine, norepinephrine, and serotonin [46, 47]. In conclusion, medications that increase the availability of these neurotransmitters may strengthen the process of neuroplasticity. The main studied medications are donepezil (cholinesterase inhibitors), memantine (noncompetitive antagonist of the Nmethyl-D-aspartate receptor), and piracetam. Preliminary positive results were found using piracetam in nonfluent aphasias (Broca's aphasia), but it has not been proven to be effective in long-term use [48].

Consequently, a series of drugs targeting improving language deficits have been studied during the last years. Until now, the conclusion is that some agents may be mainly suitable for treating speech output deficits and picture naming with poor influence over comprehension, particularly in severe cases [49]. There are some theories that support the idea that selective serotonin reuptake inhibitors (SSRIs) might be useful for persons with non-fluent aphasia (e.g., Broca's aphasia), which are also associating depression and frustration, but probably they are less suitable for persons with fluent aphasia (coursing with excitement and reduced awareness) [44].

Another promising therapeutic strategy is represented by using biotechnologically prepared peptides that stimulate neurotrophic regulation in the central nervous system (with neurotrophic and neuroprotective activities). Between 2005 and 2009, a large Romanian study has been conducted in four departments of neurology, analyzing 2212 consecutive Broca's aphasics following a first acute ischemic stroke. The purpose of this study was to evaluate the efficacy of Cerebrolysin administration (30 ml Cerebrolysin mixed with 70 ml of normal saline/day/iv infusion, for 21 days) in Broca's aphasics with acute ischemic stroke (n = 156: 52 in cerebrolysin and 104 in placebo) [50]. The conclusion of this study was that spontaneous (voluntary and automatically) speech, repetition, and naming in acute Broca's aphasia have been positive influenced [44, 50]. Our study clearly demonstrated that intravenous adjuvant treatment with cerebrolysin results in statistically significant and clinically important improvements of language function in patients with Broca's aphasia with a first acute ischemic stroke [50]. Further larger studies are crucial for sustaining this pertinent hypothesis.

5.2 Speech therapy

While pharmacological approach produces unreliable results, with small/moderate language improvements, speech therapy is nowadays considered the gold standard in recovery of aphasias. Brady et al. analyzed 57 randomized controlled trials, comparing patient group with speech therapy and other without it and demonstrated that speech therapy led to clinically significance improvements in patients' ability of communicating. The intensity and duration of speech therapy are very important, the longer the duration of therapy, the more effective the recovery [51]. In patients with chronic aphasia secondary to stroke, intensive speech and language therapy has proven superiority over delayed or even the absence of treatment [52]. Breitenstein et al. concluded that 3 weeks of intensive speech and language therapy of 10 or more hours per week can be considered an evidence-based intervention for patients with chronic aphasia after stroke (aged 70 years or younger) [52].

5.3 Transcranial magnetic stimulation (TMS)

Transcranial magnetic stimulation (TMS) is a noninvasive method of brain stimulation that relies on electromagnetic induction using an insulated coil placed over the scalp, focused on the specific, desired area of the cortex, which offers a promising alternative approach in amplifying neuroplasticity processes involved in language recovery after stroke. Repetitive transcranial magnetic stimulation (rTMS) modulates neural activity using two mechanisms: by decreasing the cortical excitability with low-frequency rTMS (⩽1 Hz) applied on nondominant hemisphere or by releasing the inhibition of the dominant hemisphere with high-frequency rTMS (⩾5 Hz).

Most trials of low-frequency or high-frequency rTMS in subacute stroke have reported significantly greater language improvement in the rTMS than in the sham group or condition [53].

Regarding rTMS in rehabilitation of Broca's aphasic patients, few studies have been conducted targeted on recovering one single type of aphasia. The meta-analysis conducted by J. Zhang and his collaborators indicated that rTMS groups had a superior language recovery than sham rTMS groups and conventional rehabilitation groups. Low-frequency rTMS brought greater improvement in language recovery (excepting comprehension) than the sham rTMS. Conversely, high-frequency rTMS did not improve the evolution of rTMS groups compared with sham rTMS and conventional rehabilitation groups (speech therapy) [54].

The entire neuroscience community is still studying different methods of stimulating the reestablishment of network connections that could finally improve language disturbances, using transcranial magnetic stimulation.

6. Conclusions

Broca'a aphasia is the third most common form of aphasia due to acute stroke. Given the severe disability suffered by aphasic patients and the complexity of language recovery (taking into consideration all forms of aphasia), studies are still insufficient to elucidate clear treatment strategies for aphasias at this time. Regarding the current clinical and imaging diagnosis, the anatomical correlations with different forms of aphasia still remain poorly understood. Several studies have demonstrated that it is possible to draw a neuroanatomical map of aphasic syndromes, which are superimposable on a significant percentage of cases reported in the literature. This concludes to the idea that the main determining factor of aphasic disorders is the neuroanatomical location of the lesion. This does not mean that the injury of one restricted area with certain language or speech functions is going to determine the same aphasic syndrome in different individuals. Examining language disturbances should focus more on aphasic symptoms rather than on aphasic syndromes.

Author details

Dragoș Cătălin Jianu[1,2,3]*, Tihomir V. Ilic[4], Silviana Nina Jianu[5], Any Docu Axelerad[6], Claudiu Dumitru Bîrdac[2,3], Traian Flavius Dan[1,2,3], Anca Elena Gogu[1,2,3] and Georgiana Munteanu[1,2,3]

1 Department of Neurosciences-Division of Neurology, Victor Babeș, University of Medicine and Pharmacy, Timisoara, Romania

2 Centre for Cognitive Research in Neuropsychiatric Pathology (NeuroPsy-Cog), Department of Neurosciences, Victor Babeș, University of Medicine and Pharmacy, Timisoara, Romania

3 First Department of Neurology, Pius Brânzeu Emergency County Hospital, Timisoara, Romania

4 Department of Neurology, Medical Faculty of Military Medical Academy, University of Defence, Belgrade, Serbia

5 Department of Ophthalmology, "Dr. Victor Popescu" Military Emergency Hospital, Timisoara, Romania

6 Department of Neurology, General Medicine Faculty, "Ovidius" University, Constanta, Romania

*Address all correspondence to: dcjianu@yahoo.com

References

[1] Ardila A. Chapter 2. Aphasia etiologies. In: Aphasia Handbook 2. Miami, Florida, USA: Florida International University; 2014. pp. 29-45

[2] Jianu DC. Elemente de afaziologie (Romanian). Mirton: Timisoara, Romania; 2001

[3] Ardila A. Chapter 4. Major aphasic syndromes: Wernicke's aphasia and Broca's aphasia. In: Aphasia Handbook 2. Miami, Florida, USA: Florida International University; 2014. pp. 60-75

[4] Pedersen PM, Vinter K, Olsen TS. Aphasia after stroke: Type, severity and prognosis. The Copenhagen aphasia study. Cerebrovascular Diseases. 2004;**17**(1):35-43. Epub 2003 Oct 3. DOI: 10.1159/000073896

[5] Abou Zeki D, Hillis A. Chapter 12. Acquired disorders of language and speech. In: Masud H, Schott JM, editors. Oxford Textbook of Cognitive Neurology and Dementia. UK: Oxford University Press; 2016. pp. 123-133

[6] Croquelois A, Godefroy O. Chapter 7. Vascular aphasias. In: Godefroy O, editor. The Behavioral and Cognitive Neurology of Stroke. 2nd ed. UK: Cambridge University Press; 2013. pp. 65-75

[7] Alajouanine T. L'aphasie et le langage pathologique. Paris: J.B. Baillière et fils éditeurs; 1968. p. 19

[8] Benson FD, Geschwind N. Aphasia and related cortical disturbances. In: Baker AB, Baker LH, editor. Clinical Neurology. Philadelphia: Harper and Row; 1971

[9] Kearns KP. Chapter 8. Broca's aphasia. In: La Pointe LL, editor. Aphasia and Related Neurogenic Language Disorders. 3rd ed. New York, Stuttgart: Thieme; 2005. pp. 117-141.

[10] Alexander MP, Naeser MA. Broca's area aphasics. Brain and Language. 1992;**43**(3):215-227

[11] Haartmann HJ, Kolk HHJ. The production of grammatical morphology in Broca's and Wernicke's aphasics. Cortex. 1992;**28**:97-112

[12] Jianu DC, Bednar M, Zolog A. Diagnosticul diferențial între tulburările fonetice şi fonologice la afazici (Romanian). Revista Societății de Neurologie şi Psihiatrie pentru Copii şi adolescenți din România. 1999;**2**:55-58

[13] Jianu DC. Managementul afazicilor romani consecutiv infarctelor cerebrale (Romanian). Mirton: Timisoara, Romania; 2011

[14] Damasio AR. Aphasia. New England Journal of Medicine. 1992;**326**:531-539

[15] Kertesz A. Clinical forms of aphasia. Acta Neurochirurgica. Supplementum (Wien). 1993;**56**:52-58

[16] Kory Calomfirescu S, Kory MM. Afazia în accidentele vasculare cerebrale (Romanian). Casa Cărții de Ştiință: Cluj-Napoca, Romania; 1996

[17] Rapp B, Goldrick M. Interactivity? The relationship between semantics and phonology in speech production. Brain and Language. 1997;**50**:1-194; 50-53

[18] Verstichel P, Cambier J. Capitolul XXVI—Afaziile. In: Botez MI, editor. Neuropsihologie clinică şi Neurologia comportamentului. Ediția a II-a ed. Masson, Editura Medicală, Bucureşti: Les Presses de L'Université de Montréal; 1996. pp. 457-491

[19] Zolog A. Afaziile, semiologie, neurolingvistică, sindromologie. Timişoara: Editura Eurobit; 1997

[20] Ardila A. Chapter 8. Associated disorders. In: Aphasia Handbook 2. Miami, Florida, USA: Florida International University; 2014. pp. 140-154

[21] Jianu DC, Jianu SN, Petrica L, Dan TF, Munteanu G. Chapter 3: Vascular aphasias. In: Ischemic Stroke. London, United Kingdom: IntechOpen; 2020. pp. 37-60. DOI: 10.5772/intechopen.92691

[22] Thompson CK. Chapter 2. Functional neuroimaging. In: La Pointe LL, editor. Aphasia and Related Neurogenic Language Disorders. 3rd ed. New York-Stuttgart: Thieme; 2005. pp. 19-38.

[23] Hanna D. Chapter I. Neuroimaging contributions to the understanding of aphasia. In: Boller F, editor. Handbook of Neuropsychology. Vol. 2. Amsterdam, Netherlands: Elsevier Science Publishers, B.V; 1989

[24] Poeck K, de Bleser R, von Keyserlink DG. Computed tomography localization of standard aphasic syndromes. In: Rose FC, editor. Advances in Neurology. Vol. 42. Progress in Aphasiology. New York: Raven Press; 1984. pp. 71-89

[25] Kreisler A, Goderfroy O, Delmaire C. The anatomy of aphasia revisited. Neurology. 2000;**54**:1117-1123

[26] Godefroy O, Dubois C, Debachy B, et al. Vascular aphasias main characteristics of patients hospitalized in acute stroke units. Stroke. 2002;**33**: 702-706

[27] Yang Z-H, Zhao X-Q, Wang C-X, Chenand H-Y, Zhang Y-M. Neuroanatomic correlation of the post-stroke aphasias studied with imaging. Neurological Research. 2008;**30**:356-360. DOI: 10.1179/174313208X300332

[28] Basso A, Lecours AR, Moraschini S, et al. Anatomoclinical correlations of the aphasias as defined through computerized tomography: Exceptions. Brain and Language. 1985;**26**:201-229

[29] Willmes K, Poeck K. To what extent can aphasic syndromes be localized? Brain. 1993;**116**:1527-1540

[30] Nina F, Dronkers A. The pursuit of brain–language relationships. Brain and Language. 2000;**71**:59-61

[31] Hallowell B. Aphasia and Other Acquired Neurogenic Language Disorders: A Guide Forclinical Excellence. San Diego, CA: Plural Publishing; 2017. Chapter 8. pp. 122-124. ISBN 9781597564779

[32] Ropper AH, Brown RH. Chapter 23: Disorders of speech and language. In: Adams and Victor's Victor's Principles of Neurology. 8th edition. New York: Mc Graw-Hill; 2005. pp. 413-430

[33] Damasio AR. The neural basis of language. Annual Review of Neuroscience (Palo Alto, CA). 1984;**7**:127-147

[34] Caplan LR et al. Caudate infarcts. Archives of Neurology. 1990;**47**:133-143

[35] Demeurisse G, Demol O, Beuckelaer RDE. Quantitative study of the rate of recovery from aphasia due to ischemic stroke. Stroke. 1979;**11**(5): 455-458

[36] Kertesz A, Mccabe P. Recovery patterns and prognosis in aphasia. Brain. 1977;**100**:1-18

[37] Mazzoni M, Vista M, Pardossi L, Avila L, et al. Spontaneous evolution of aphasia after ischaemic stroke. Aphasiology. 1992;**6**(4):37-41

[38] Basso A, Capitani E, Vignolo LA. Influence of rehabilitation on language skills in aphasic patients. A controlled study. Archives of Neurology. 1979; **36**(4):190-196

[39] El Hachioui H, Lingsma HF, van de Sandt-Koenderman ME, Dippel DWJ, Koudstaal PJ, Visch-Brink EG. Recovery of aphasia after stroke: A 1-year follow-up study. Journal of Neurology. 2013;**260**(1):166-171

[40] NINDS TPA (The National Institute of Neurological Disorders and Stroke RT-PA Stroke Study Group). Tissue plasminogen activator for acute ischemic stroke. The New England Journal of Medicine. 1995;**333**:1581-1587

[41] Campbell BCV, Mitchell PJ, Kleinig TJ, et al. Endovascular therapy for ischemic stroke with perfusion-imaging selection. The New England Journal of Medicine. 2015;**372**:1009-1018

[42] Crijnen YS, Nouwens F, de Lau LML, et al. Early effect of intra-arterial treatment in ischemic stroke on aphasia recovery in MR CLEAN. Neurology. 2016;**86**:2049-2055

[43] Hillis AE, Ulatowski JA, Barker PB, et al. A pilot randomized trial of induced blood pressure elevation: Effects on function and focal perfusion in acute and subacute stroke. Cerebrovascular Diseases. 2003;**16**:236-246

[44] Berthier ML. Ten key reasons for continuing research on pharmacotherapy for post-stroke aphasia. Aphasiology. 2021;**35**(6):824-858

[45] Crosson B, Rodriguez AD, Copland D, et al. Neuroplasticity and aphasia treatments: New approaches for an old problem. Journal of Neurology, Neurosurgery, and Psychiatry. 2019;**90**: 1147-1155

[46] Brzosko Z, Mierau SB, Paulsen O. Neuromodulation of spike-timing-dependent plasticity: Past, present, and future. Neuron. 2019;**103**:563-581

[47] Llano DA, Small SL. Pharmacotherapy for Aphasia. In: Small S, Hickok G, editors. Neurobiology of Language. Amsterdam: Elsevier; 2015. pp. 1067-1083

[48] Güngör L, Terzi M, Onar MK. Does long term use of piracetam improve speech disturbances due to ischemic cerebrovascular diseases? Brain and Language. 2011;**117**:23-27

[49] Woodhead ZV, Crinion J, Teki S, Penny W, Price CJ, Leff AP. Auditory training changes temporal lobe connectivity in 'Wernicke's aphasia': A randomised trial. Journal of Neurology, Neurosurgery, and Psychiatry. 2017; **88**(7):586-594. DOI: 10.1136/jnnp-2016-314621

[50] Jianu DC, Muresanu DF, Bajenaru O, Popescu BO, Deme SM, Moessler H, et al. Cerebrolysin adjuvant treatment in Broca's aphasics following first acute ischemic stroke of the left middle cerebral artery. Journal of Medicine and Life. 2010;**3**(3):297-307

[51] Brady MC, Kelly H, Godwin J, Enderby P, Campbell P. Speech and language therapy for aphasia following stroke. Cochrane Database of Systematic Reviews. 2016;**6**:CD000425

[52] Breitenstein C, Grewe T, Flöel A, Ziegler W, Springer L, Martus P, et al. Intensive speech and language therapy in patients with chronic aphasia after stroke: A randomised, open-label, blinded-endpoint, controlled trial in a health-care setting. Lancet. 2017;**389**(10078):1528-1538. Epub 2017 Mar 1. Erratum in: Lancet. 2017;**389**(10078):1518

[53] Tsai P-Y, Wang C-P, Ko JS, Chung Y-M, Chang Y-W, Wang J-X. The persistent and broadly modulating effect of inhibitory rTMS in nonfluent aphasic patients: A sham-controlled, double-blind study. Neurorehabilitation and Neural Repair. 2014;**28**:779-787

[54] Zhang J, Zhong D, Xiao X, Yuan L, Li Y, Zheng Y, et al. Effects of repetitive transcranial magnetic stimulation (rTMS) on aphasia in stroke patients: A systematic review and meta-analysis. Clinical Rehabilitation. 2021;**35**(8):1103-11116. DOI: 10.1177/0269215521999554

Chapter 3

Imaging of Vascular Aphasia

Loïc Duron, Augustin Lecler, Dragoș Cătălin Jianu, Raphaël Sadik and Julien Savatovsky

Abstract

Brain imaging is essential for the diagnosis of acute stroke and vascular aphasia. Magnetic resonance imaging (MRI) is the modality of choice for the etiological diagnosis of aphasia, the assessment of its severity, and the prediction of recovery. Diffusion weighted imaging is used to detect, localize, and quantify the extension of the irreversibly injured brain tissue called ischemic core. Perfusion weighted imaging (from MRI or CT) is useful to assess the extension of hypoperfused but salvageable tissue called penumbra. Functional imaging (positron emission tomography (PET), functional MRI (fMRI)) may help predicting recovery and is useful for the understanding of language networks and individual variability. This chapter is meant to review the state of the art of morphological and functional imaging of vascular aphasia and to illustrate the MRI profiles of different aphasic syndromes.

Keywords: aphasia, stroke, imaging, MRI, recovery

1. Introduction

Aphasia is an acquired language disorder caused by damage to language regions of the brain that can affect the ability of a person to understand and/or produce language. It is often accompanied by impairment in reading (alexia) and writing (agraphia). Aphasia is one of the most common and debilitating consequences of stroke and is associated with a higher risk of mortality, a poor functional prognosis, and an augmented risk of vascular dementia. Fortunately, some degree of recovery of language function occurs for about 70% of patients with post-stroke aphasia thanks to neural plasticity and speech and language therapy [1–3].

Brain imaging is essential for the initial diagnosis of stroke and the assessment of stroke severity and prognosis. Stroke location and extension are associated with different patterns of aphasia with diverse functional outcomes [2]. Functional imaging, such as positron emission tomography (PET), functional magnetic resonance imaging (fMRI), and magnetoencephalography (MEG), has also been extensively evaluated for its ability to predict recovery from aphasia [4].

The purpose of this chapter is to review the state of the art of morphological and functional imaging of vascular aphasia and to illustrate the MRI profiles of different aphasic syndromes.

2. Brain language areas

Aphasia is caused by a brain damage localized in one or several language areas of the left hemisphere for 95% of right-handed people and 75% of left-handed

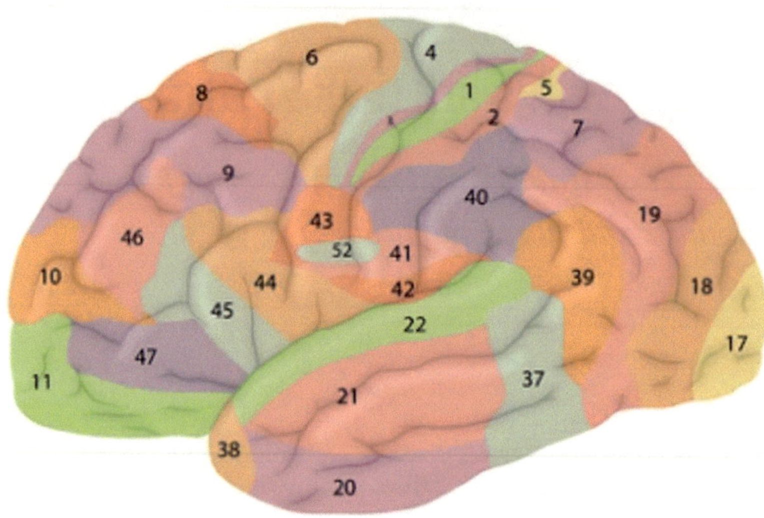

Figure 1.
Lateral view of Brodmann areas.

people. Functional neuroimaging techniques have highlighted Brodman Areas (BA, **Figure 1**) associated with language functions. They are clustered into two main language networks: (1) a language reception/understanding system, including a "core Wernicke's area" involved in word recognition (BA21, BA22, BA41, and BA42), and a peripheral area ("extended Wernicke's area:" BA20, BA37, BA38, BA39, and BA40) involved in language associations; (2) a language production system ("Broca's complex:" BA44, BA45, and also BA46, BA47, partially BA6—mainly its mesial supplementary motor area—and extending toward the basal ganglia and the thalamus. The insula (BA13) may also play a coordinating role in interconnecting these two brain language networks [5–7].

A given language impairment can result from damage or dysfunction of several different brain areas due to the impact of the lesion not only on the function of the affected region but also on the many regions connected to it within the language networks.

3. Imaging of aphasia

Brain imaging is critical to the initial management of ischemic stroke. Magnetic Resonance (MR) diffusion and perfusion imaging as well as computed tomography (CT) perfusion imaging are commonly used in clinical routine for estimation of ischemic core, penumbra, outcome prediction, and treatment decision-making in the acute stroke setting. Functional MRI is used after the initial phase to assess the severity of aphasia and predict recovery.

3.1 Ischemic core

The ischemic core corresponds to brain tissue that has been irreversibly injured and has already turned or will inevitably turn into infarction regardless of treatment [8]. It can be assessed on non-contrast CT as hypo-attenuating areas and on Diffusion Weighted Imaging (DWI) of MRI exams as hyperintense areas with decreased Apparent Diffusion Coefficient (ADC) values on ADC map. The ischemic core can also be assessed using CT or MR perfusion imaging and is currently defined as areas with relative Cerebral Blood Flow (CBF) < 30% compared with the baseline level. However, hyperintense lesions on DWI, hypodense areas on CT, and areas with CBF < 30% on perfusion CT or MRI can be partially reversible, particularly if reperfusion is performed within 30 min, so that there is no gold standard for ischemic core imaging.

3.2 Penumbra

The ischemic penumbra is defined as an area of nonfunctioning but viable brain tissue that may recover its function if blood flow is restored. Therefore, it is the main target of reperfusion treatments. The ischemic penumbra has been widely investigated because of its potential to personalize therapeutic opportunities. It can be assessed using CT or MR perfusion and is defined as the area outside the ischemic core with a time-to-maximum (Tmax) > 6 s (**Figure 2**). A large area of penumbra associated with a small ischemic core represents a good candidate for reperfusion therapeutics such as intravenous thrombolysis and mechanical thrombectomy. This reperfusion is highly correlated with improvements on specific language tasks [1].

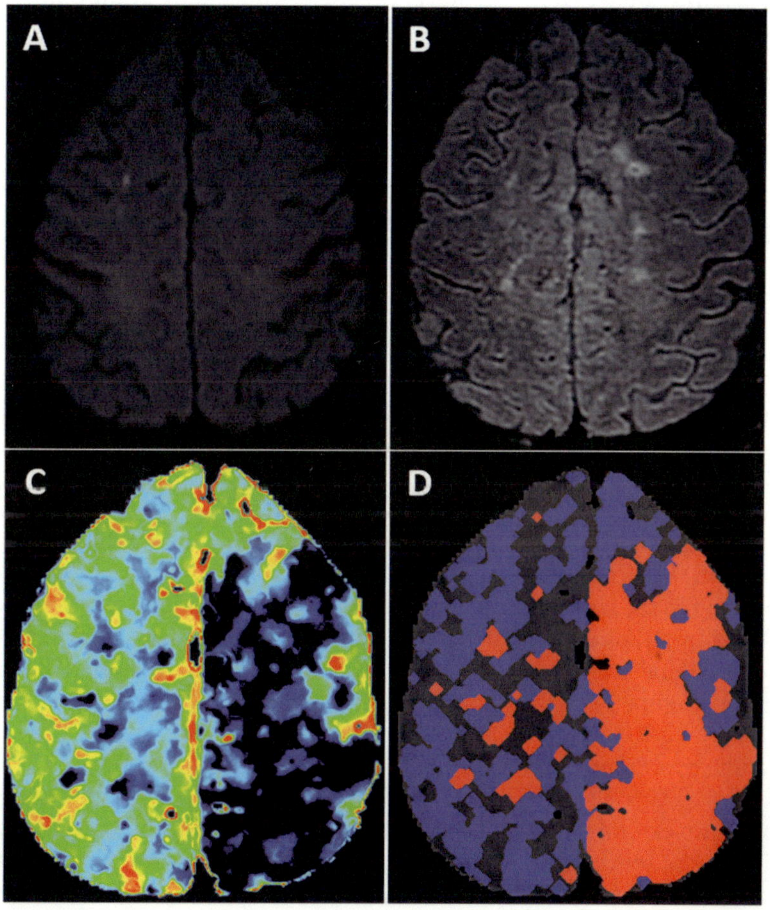

Figure 2.
Left sylvian acute ischemic stroke in a 44-year-old man with global aphasia. DWI (A) and FLAIR (B) are normal in the left sylvian area and show an isolated ischemic spot in the right sylvian area. Perfusion maps show a decrease in cerebral blood flow (C, dark blue) in the left sylvian area, with a consistent increase in Tmax > 6 s (D, red). This corresponds to ischemic penumbra, i.e., salvageable tissue that may benefit from reperfusion treatments.

3.3 Recovery prediction

Depending on the location and extent of the left hemisphere lesion, different mechanisms may concur to recovery from aphasia: (1) right hemisphere reorganization, (2) implication of residual left hemisphere language areas, (3) recruitment of left hemisphere regions not previously involved in language function, and (4) reorientation of domain-general networks not specifically dedicated to language [1, 9–11]. Intensive and targeted language therapy may interact with brain plasticity to favor recovery from aphasia.

Several neuroimaging findings were associated with aphasia severity and poor recovery, such as a large volume of ischemia, a cortical involvement, a non-fluent profile of aphasia, and a high National Institutes of Health Stroke Scale (NIHSS) score at 2 weeks [12].

Functional imaging has also been extensively investigated for its potential to predict recovery from aphasia. However, the generalizability, variability, and interpretability of group-based approaches that most imaging studies use have been criticized because of the variability in mapping function onto macro-anatomy across neurologically healthy individuals, which hinders the interpretation of results at the individual level. Therefore, the methods used in studies must be carefully validated to safely generalize the findings [13].

4. Illustration of aphasic syndromes

The location and extension of the stroke lesions are the main determinants of the aphasic profile. Eight patterns of aphasia will be illustrated below: Broca's aphasia, Wernicke's aphasia, conduction, transcortical, global, anomic, crossed, and subcortical aphasia.

4.1 Broca's aphasia

Broca's aphasia is generally produced by infarcts or severe hypoperfusion of the superior division of the left middle cerebral artery [2, 14, 15]. Brain areas involved in Broca's aphasia are classically:

1. Broca's area: the posterior part of the third frontal gyrus—BA44 and BA45. Lesions in this area determine transitory apraxia of speech. Larger lesions, extending to the subjacent white matter, produce transitory mutism, which is replaced by a rapidly improving syndrome with prominent arthric deformations and deficits in action naming that are more severe than deficits in object naming (**Figure 3**).

2. Rolandic operculum: lower part of motor area: Fa (**Figure 4**).

3. Lesions can extend or separately affect insular cortex (**Figure 5**) and subjacent white matter, centrum semi-ovale, capsule-striatum (caudate nucleus head and putamen), and periventricular areas. Infarctions involving together these structures and Broca's area may also produce the complete syndrome of Broca's aphasia.

4.2 Wernicke's aphasia

Wernicke aphasia is generally produced by infarcts or severe hypoperfusion of the inferior division of the left middle cerebral artery, which supplies the posterior

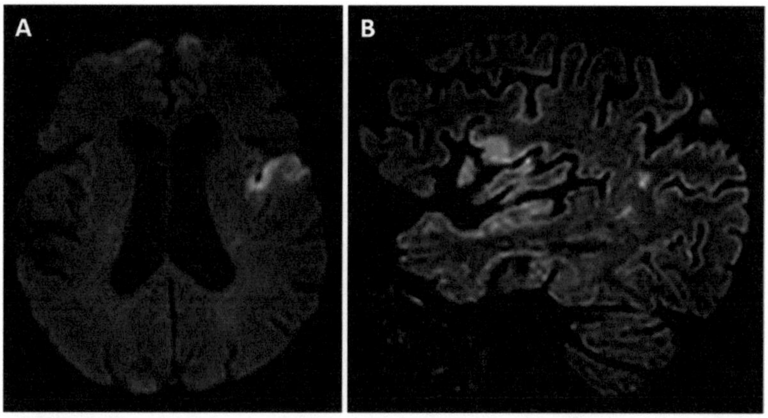

Figure 3.
Broca and left Rolandic operculum acute ischemic stroke in a 65-year-old woman presenting with Broca's aphasia, hyperintense on DWI (A) and FLAIR (B).

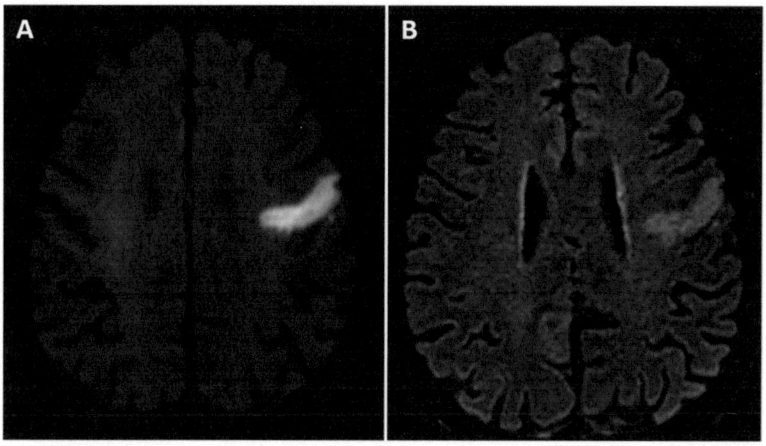

Figure 4.
Left inferior frontal gyrus acute ischemic stroke in a 82-year-old man presenting with Broca's aphasia, hyperintense on DWI (A) and FLAIR (B).

part of the temporal lobe and inferior parietal lobule [2, 14, 15]. Brain areas involved in Wernicke's aphasia are classically:

1. Wernicke's area: posterior part of the first two temporal gyri-T1/T2 (BA22) (**Figure 6**).

2. Inferior parietal lobes: angular gyrus (BA39) and supramarginal gyrus (BA40).

3. Lesions can extend to the insular-external capsule region and anterior part of temporal gyri (BA22). Besides the cortical destructions from these areas, subjacent white matter can be also affected.

4.3 Conduction aphasia

The lesions affect the inferior parietal lobes, especially the supramarginal gyrus and/or the external capsule; they classically disrupt the arcuate fasciculus, although its role remains debated for the repetition impairments: probably

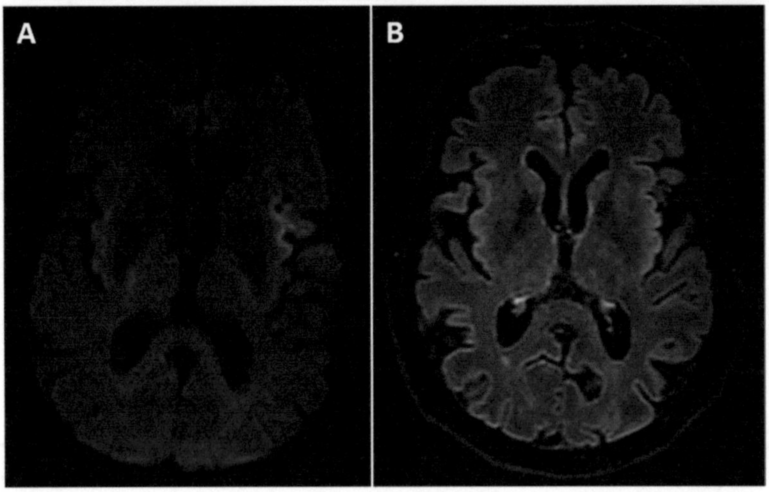

Figure 5.
Acute ischemic stroke of the left insula in a 62-year-old man with hyperacute Broca's aphasia, hyperintense on DWI (A) but still normal on FLAIR (B).

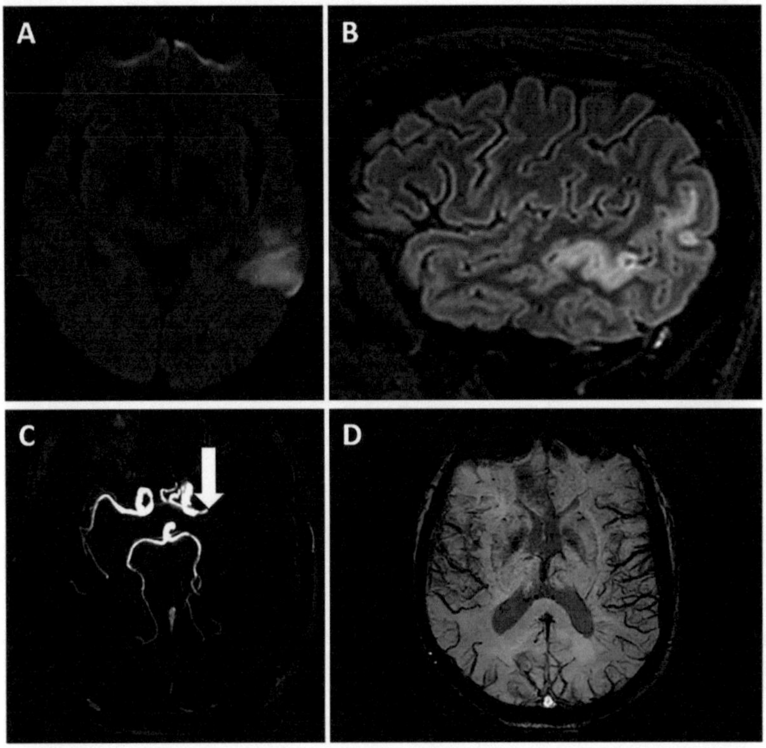

Figure 6.
Acute ischemic stroke of the left temporal gyri in a 63-year-old man presenting with acute Wernicke's aphasia, hyperintense on DWI (A) and FLAIR (B). The left middle cerebral artery is occluded (C, arrow). Dilated cortical veins are visible in the larger hypoperfused area (D), known as "cortical brush sign."

disconnection between the superior temporal cortex and the inferior frontal gyri, respectively [2, 14, 15].

Other explanations for the repetition impairments have been noted, such as short-term memory syndrome (the repetition impairment due to limited working

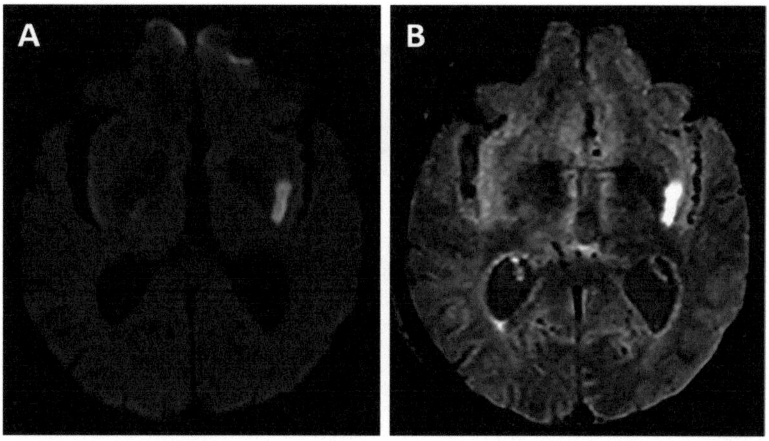

Figure 7.
Acute ischemic stroke of the left external capsule in a 88-year-old man presenting with conduction aphasia, hyperintense on DWI (A) and FLAIR (B).

memory)—so, the associated lesions are situated in areas critical for working memory: inferior parietal lobule (supramarginal and angular gyri), inferior frontal cortex, posterior temporal lobe, and/or their white matter connections (the external capsule (**Figure 7**).

Conduction aphasia is the result of an embolic infarct of the inferior division (posterior temporal or parietal) of the left middle cerebral artery. It is rarely observed at the acute stage of stroke and more frequently affects younger patients [16].

4.4 Transcortical aphasias

Cortical lesions isolating the spared peri-sylvian language areas (watershed territory between the left anterior cerebral artery and middle cerebral artery in addition to the watershed territory between the left middle cerebral artery and posterior cerebral artery).

Subcortical lesions: large thalamic hemorrhage interrupting the temporal isthmus; infarcts in the left thalamus, putamen, and periventricular white matter [17].

4.5 Global aphasia

Extended lesions (including left peri-sylvian anterior and posterior language areas), which are the result of a left middle cerebral artery or carotid artery occlusion (with a total left middle cerebral artery infarct), produce global aphasia with hemiplegia, hemisensory deficits, and hemianopia [2, 14, 15].

Broca's and Wernicke's areas may be simultaneously hypoperfused in the acute period. Thus, global aphasia can be the initial aphasic syndrome (**Figure 8**).

Early involution into Broca's aphasia (with early recovery of comprehension) may result from reperfusion of Wernicke's area. In this case, the patient presents only left frontal lobe, left basal ganglia, and left insula ischemic lesions (diffusion-weighted image shows infarct in superior division of left middle cerebral artery territory, which includes Broca's area), sparing in the same time the left temporo-parietal region (global aphasia with hemiplegia and early improvement of comprehension). Later recovery of comprehension may appear from the reorganization of the language network:

- Frontal and temporoparietal lesions (two lesions) produce global aphasia without hemiplegia. When sensory-motor deficit is missing, we should search for mixed transcortical aphasia.
- Subcortical infarct extended into basal ganglia.

4.6 Anomic aphasia

Acute anomic aphasia may be noted after stroke in many locations. It also represents a stage of all aphasic syndromes when they improve.

4.7 Crossed aphasias

This is a very rare condition (1% of all acute ischemic stroke aphasias), defined by an aphasic syndrome in a right-handed patient (free from developmental disorders and previous brain lesions, fully lateralized, which is demonstrated using a questionnaire such as Edinburgh Inventory), caused by a right hemisphere lesion (non-dominant hemisphere) [2, 14, 15].

The anatomical determinants are similar to those observed in left hemisphere lesion, although a higher proportion of deviant cases are observed, particularly with mild aphasia contrasting with the large lesion. This fact is usually reported as evidence

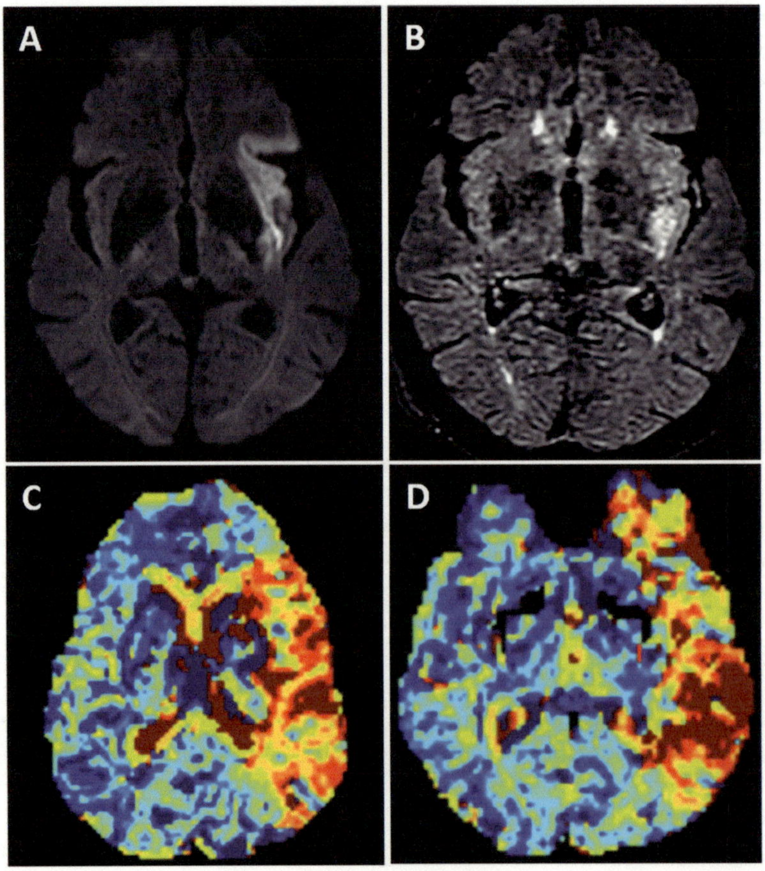

Figure 8.
Acute ischemic stroke of the left sylvian territory in a 76-year-old man with ischemic core involving the Broca's area on DWI (A) and FLAIR (B) and penumbra involving the Wernicke's area (C and D). Global aphasia improved after recanalization, resulting in a chronic non-fluent Broca's aphasia.

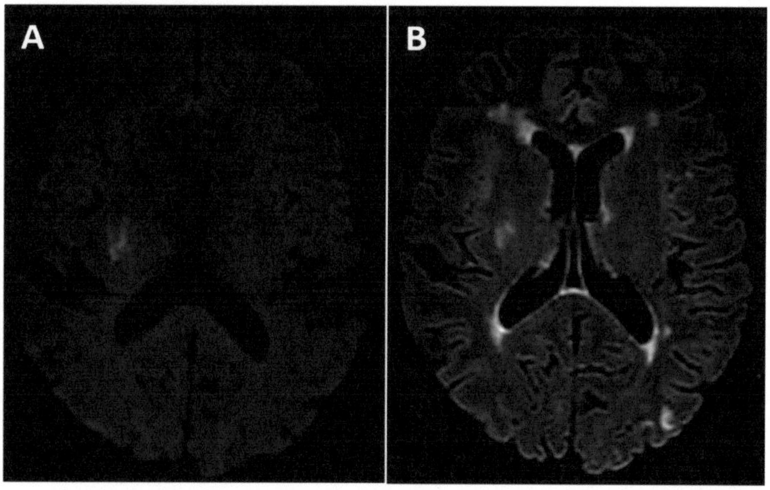

Figure 9.
Acute ischemic stroke of the right external capsule in a 76-year-old man presenting with global aphasia, hyperintense on DWI (A) and FLAIR (B).

for bilateral representation of the language. In the past, crossed aphasia was considered to be non-fluent, although today is reported that all aphasic syndromes can be registered (some cases of crossed Wernicke's aphasia in right-handed patients with lesions in the homologous area of the right cerebral hemisphere are noted) (**Figure 9**).

4.8 Subcortical aphasias

Pure left striato-capsular infarcts (left deep middle cerebral artery infarcts) can produce different types of aphasias (mainly non-fluent, especially motor transcortical aphasia and Broca's aphasia) (**Figure 10**). Frequently, hypophonia (poor speech volume) can be noted [2, 14, 15].

Fluent and non-fluent aphasias have been reported in thalamic lesions. Usually, a thalamic aphasia presents a significant impairment of spontaneous speech, with verbal paraphasias, but with oral comprehension and repetition relatively spared [1, 2, 5]. Patients with subcortical aphasias are older, because the main mechanism of ischemic stroke is small vascular disease.

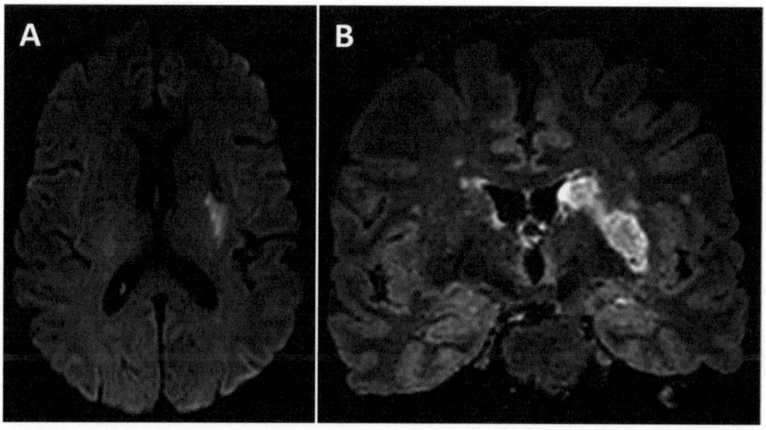

Figure 10.
Acute ischemic stroke of the left striato-capsular area in a 66-year-old woman with subcortical aphasia, hyperintense on DWI (A) and FLAIR (B).

There are two distinct mechanisms concerning subcortical vascular aphasias: (a) a possible sustained cortical hypoperfusion and infarction not visible on structural imaging studies and (b) a possible thalamic disconnection, due to striato-capsular infarcts.

5. Conclusions

Brain imaging, especially MRI, is the cornerstone of the etiological diagnosis and prognostic evaluation of vascular aphasia. Location and extent of the ischemic core are valuable information to assess the severity of aphasia and predict recovery. Despite overlap in MRI patterns between aphasic syndromes, two main networks are known to induce specific language deficit: the anterior network centered on the Broca's area and the posterior network centered on the Wernicke's area. Perfusion imaging is helpful to determine the mismatch between irreversibly injured tissue in the ischemic core and salvageable tissue in the ischemic penumbra that may benefit from reperfusion treatment and result in symptoms recovery.

Future work may focus on the discovery of new imaging biomarkers to help predict aphasia recovery with better accuracy and orient specific treatments.

Acknowledgements

The authorship criteria are listed in our Authorship Policy: https://www.intechopen.com/page/authorship-policy. This section of your manuscript may also include funding information.

Conflict of interest

The authors declare no conflict of interest.

Author details

Loïc Duron[1*], Augustin Lecler[1], Dragoş Cătălin Jianu[2], Raphaël Sadik[3] and Julien Savatovsky[1]

1 Department of Radiology, Foundation Rothschild Hospital, Paris, France

2 Department of Neurology, "Victor Babes" University of Medicine and Pharmacy, Timisoara, Romania

3 Foundation Rothschild Hospital, Paris, France

*Address all correspondence to: lduron@for.paris

References

[1] Thompson CK, den Ouden DB. Neuroimaging and recovery of language in aphasia. Current Neurology and Neuroscience Reports. 2008;**8**(6):475-483

[2] Abou Zeki D, Hillis A. Chapter 12. Acquired disorders of language and speech. In: Masud H, Schott JM, editors. Oxford Textbook of Cognitive Neurology and Dementia. UK: Oxford University Press; 2016. pp. 123-133

[3] Croquelois A, Godefroy O. Vascular aphasias. In: Godefroy O, editor. The Behavioral and Cognitive Neurology of Stroke. Cambridge: Cambridge University Press; 2013. pp. 65-75

[4] Rosenberg MD, Song H. Predicting post-stroke aphasia from brain imaging. Nature Human Behaviour. 2020; **4**:675-676

[5] Ardila A, Bernal B, Rosselli M. How localized are language brain areas? A review of brodmann areas involvement in oral language. Archives of Clinical Neuropsychology. 2016;**31**(1):112-122

[6] Fridriksson J, den Ouden D-B, Hillis AE, Hickok G, Rorden C, Basilakos A, et al. Anatomy of aphasia revisited. Brain: A Journal of Neurology. 2018;**141**(3):848-862

[7] Jiménez de la Peña MM, Gómez Vicente L, García Cobos R, Martínez de Vega V. Neuroradiologic correlation with aphasias. Cortico-subcortical map of language. Radiología. 2018;**60**(3): 250-261

[8] Goyal M, Ospel JM, Menon B, Almekhlafi M, Jayaraman M, Fiehler J, et al. Challenging the ischemic core concept in acute ischemic stroke imaging. Stroke. 2020;**51**(10):3147-3155

[9] Stephen MW, Schneck SM. Neuroplasticity in post-stroke aphasia: A systematic review and meta-analysis of functional imaging studies of reorganization of language processing. Neurobiology of Language. 2021;**2**(1): 22-82

[10] Lorca-Puls DL, Gajardo-Vidal A, PLORAS Team, Oberhuber M, Prejawa S, TMH H, et al. Brain regions that support accurate speech production after damage to Broca's area. Brain Communications. 2021;**3**(4):fcab230

[11] Chen X, Chen L, Zheng S, Wang H, Dai Y, Chen Z, et al. Disrupted brain connectivity networks in aphasia revealed by resting-state fMRI. Frontiers in Aging Neuroscience. 2021;**13**:666301

[12] Lee S, Na Y, Tae W-S, Pyun S-B. Clinical and neuroimaging factors associated with aphasia severity in stroke patients: diffusion tensor imaging study. Scientific Reports. 2020;**10**(1):12874

[13] Blank IA, Kiran S, Fedorenko E. Can neuroimaging help aphasia researchers? Addressing generalizability, variability, and interpretability. Cognitive Neuropsychology. 2017;**34**(6):377-393

[14] Lapointe L, Sierwalt J. Aphasia and related neurogenic language disorders. New York: Thieme; 2018

[15] Sebastian R, Breining B. Contributions of neuroimaging to understanding language deficits in acute stroke. Seminars in Speech and Language. 2018;**39**:066-078

[16] Benson DF, Sheremata WA, Bouchard R, Segarra JM, Price D, Geschwind N. Conduction aphasia. A clinicopathological study. Archives of Neurology. 1973;**28**(5):339-346

[17] Maeshima S, Osawa A. Thalamic lesions and aphasia or neglect. Current Neurology and Neuroscience Reports. 2018;**18**(7):39

Chapter 4

Primary Progressive Aphasia (PPA)

Yashaswini Channabasave Gowda and Hema Nagaraj

Abstract

Primary progressive aphasia (PPA) is a rare neurological condition that affects an individual's ability to communicate. PPA is a syndrome characterized by a 'progressive worsening of language with preservation of the activities of daily living and evidence of relatively normal non-verbal abilities on neuropsychological testing'. It commonly appears initially as a disorder of speaking (an articulatory problem) progressing to nearly total inability to speak in its most severe stage, while comprehension remains relatively preserved. This chapter provides an overview of the characteristic features of PPA, its classification, assessment, and rehabilitation options.

Keywords: Primary Progressive Aphasia, neurology, speech-language, dementia, assessment, management

1. Introduction

Primary Progressive Aphasia (PPA) is a type of dementia characterized by a loss in one or more language functions in people under the age of 65 (and occasionally as early as the 40's). It is a type of dementia and the condition is caused due to degeneration of nerve cells in the brain which control our ability to communicate [1].

PPA is a condition marked by a steady deterioration of language skills while maintaining everyday activities and showing relatively normal nonverbal abilities in neuropsychological testing. It frequently begins as a speech deficit (an articulatory problem), advancing to near total inability to speak in its most severe stage, but understanding remains largely intact.

Other neurological illnesses, on the other hand, exist in which language degeneration is simply one aspect of a broader, progressive decrease in mental processes such as memory, attention, visuospatial skills, reasoning, and the ability to perform complicated physical activities. The generation of phonemic paraphasias in naming was offered as a further criterion for separating PPA from progressive aphasia in likely Alzheimer's disease [2].

2. A retrospective delineation

Pick [3] described a patient who had a progressive language disorder that was linked to left temporal lobe atrophy. This seminal paper was followed by a flood of cases [1, 2], and it became clear that PPA can present in both fluent and non-fluent people. Over the next few decades, there were intermittent incidents [1, 4].

Mesulam's describes PPA in the context of atrophy seen in the left focal perisylvian region or temporal lobe [5]. Speech is grammatically structured and well-articulated but gradually loses content words.

The study of patients with a progressive deficit in semantic memory began at the same time as the study of cognitive issues linked with neurodegenerative disease [6, 7]. The rising anomia exhibited in these people, according to Warrington, was caused by a fundamental loss of semantic memory, which impaired object recognition and knowledge, as well as word discovery and comprehension. Following more evidence of impaired nonverbal conceptual understanding (semantic memory) as well as anomia in these patients, the term 'SD' was coined. The 1998 consensus declaration is often quoted. Associative agnosia (difficulty recognizing/identifying items) and/or prosopagnosia (difficulty recognizing/identifying known or renowned individuals) were supported as criterion for SD in the widely recognized 1998 consensus statement. PPA is currently included in the frontotemporal lobar degeneration, frontotemporal dementia, Pick's disease, or Pick's complex family of disorders.

3. Characteristics of PPA

Main characteristics of PPA [8] are as follows:

- Age of onset ranges from 40 to 75, with a mean of 59.3 years.

- The involvement of males predominates over females, with the ratio of 2:1.

- The duration of isolated language symptoms can range from 1 to 15 years with a mean of 5.3 years.

- Autopsy findings reported for 14 cases disclosed; Pick's a disease in 4, Creutzfeld—Jakob's disease in 3, Alzheimer's disease in 3, focal spongiform degeneration in 2, and nonspecific cellular changes in 2. The diversity of pathology does not support the existence of a specific disease underlying isolated language decline.

- Of the 47 cases with CT scan, 13 were normal, 5 showed a diffuse abnormality, 10 had greater left than right abnormality, and 19 had left hemisphere abnormality only.

- Most of the reported cases had predominantly fluent, anomic, or Wernicke's like aphasia, but 12 cases with nonfluent or Broca's aphasia have been described.

- The description of cases with PPA has aided in the long-running, more general debate over whether a stage model or a subgroup model [9] might be more appropriate for explaining the neuropsychological consequences of certain degenerative brain diseases, as they appeared to support a subgroup model.

- Subgroup models do not presume that cognitive performance is disintegrated uniformly. Rather, they assume that observed disparities between patients and patient groups are qualitative in origin and represent impairments in various cognitive modules.

- Stage models, on the other hand, assume a global progression of cognitive deficiencies with solely quantitative changes over time, with observed disparities between patients and patient groups explained by distinct points on a one-dimensional time-axis.

Early symptoms:

- Difficulties recalling the names of people and objects,
- Difficulties expressing one's thoughts orally and sometimes difficulty understanding others.
- Memory of recent events, attention/concentration, judgment and reasoning abilities, and visuospatial abilities are relatively normal.
- Some patients tend to say or nod "yes" for "no" and vice versa.
- Gradual difficulty in one or more of the following language functions like speaking, understanding, reading and writing.
- Inability to follow conversations or verbal instructions.
- Inability to read or write a letter.
- Decreasing content in speech or garbled speech to eventually becoming mute.

Later symptoms:

- As PPA progresses, it becomes increasingly difficult to communicate verbally by any means.
- The capacity to comprehend what others are saying or reading deteriorates as well.
- Inability to understand speech.
- Difficulty following conversations, especially in bigger groups.
- Requesting information to be repeated and misinterpreting what is said despite normal hearing.
- Early in the course of the illness, speech may become empty of any genuine information and difficult to grasp.
- Eventually, speech may be unable to communicate, leading to muteness.
- Math and calculating problems.
- Loss of ability to do even elementary mathematical processes.

Diagnostic criteria for PPA [10]:

- A distinctive feature is an insidious onset and slow advancement of word-finding, object naming, or word understanding as shown during spontaneous conversation or as tested through formal neuropsychological language tests.

- For at least 2 years following, the language impairment is responsible for all limitations in daily living activities.
- Premorbid linguistic function is intact (except for developmental dyslexia).
- Within the first 2 years of the illness, there was no notable apathy, disinhibition, forgetfulness for recent events, visuospatial impairment, visual recognition deficiencies, or sensory-motor dysfunction.
- Even in the first 2 years, acalculia and ideomotor apraxia may be present (mild constructional deficits and perseveration are also acceptable as long as neither visuospatial deficits nor disinhibition influence daily living activities).
- Other domains may be impacted after the first 2 years, but the language remains the most impaired function and deteriorates quicker than other afflicted domains throughout the illness.
- Neuroimaging has revealed that there are no "particular" reasons such as stroke or tumor.

4. Types of Primary Progressive Aphasia

The **most common type** of brain degeneration found after brain autopsy in individuals with PPA (60% of cases) is *Nonspecific degeneration (NSD)* where there is evidence of brain cell death, but no features of Alzheimer's or Pick's disease. Less commonly, Pick or Alzheimer's disease may be found.

Primary progressive aphasia, or PPA, is a group of Fronto-Temporal Dementia (FTD) symptoms defined by a progressive loss of capacity to talk, read, write, and understand what others are saying. When the following three conditions are met, PPA is diagnosed:

1. There is a steady deterioration in verbal ability (not just speech).
2. At first, the sole disability is a linguistic barrier.
3. A neurological illness is the root reason.

PPA is further divided into three clinical subgroups based on the language abilities that are most impacted, according to experts.

4.1 Semantic variant of PPA

The increasing loss of word meanings is a feature of semantic variant PPA (svPPA). The disorder is sometimes known as semantic dementia if there are extra substantial issues recognizing things or faces. Other language skills remain unchanged, such as the ability to make speech and repeat words and sentences uttered by others. However, while the affected person may continue to speak fluently, their speech becomes hazy and difficult to comprehend due to the omission or substitution of several words. People with svPPA (also known as PPA-S) may demonstrate changes in behavior compared to those seen in behavioral variant of Fronto-Temporal Dementia (bvFTD), such as disinhibition and rigid food preferences, as the disorder progresses.

Signs and symptoms:

- **Anomia**—An inability to recall the names of objects; difficulty "finding the right word." ("car" for "truck.")

- **Reduced single-word comprehension**—The person affected is unable to recall what words mean, especially words that are less familiar or less frequently used.

- **Impaired object knowledge**—Being unable to remember what a familiar object is or how it is used.

- **Surface dyslexia/dysgraphia**—Reading and writing words that do not follow standard pronunciation or spelling conventions can be difficult; such words are spelled or spoken "as if" they do. For example, the person might write "no" instead of "know" or misread "wide" as "broad."

4.2 Non-fluent variant of PPA

People with the non-fluent/agrammatic form of PPA (nfvPPA, also known as PPA-G), also known as progressive non-fluent aphasia or PNFA, have trouble speaking but, can remember the meanings of individual words. Degeneration of the areas of the brain that regulate specific linked muscles causes them to lose their ability to make sounds with their lips and tongue; nevertheless, the muscles themselves are intact. Apraxia of speech is the technical term for these issues (AOS). As a result, their speech becomes labored and slow, and they may appear to be physically struggling to speak. However, speech issues alone are not enough to diagnose PPA. When speech rather than language is the primary difficulty, the diagnosis is progressive AOS rather than PPA. The impairment of grammar is a distinctive characteristic. When speaking, people with nfvPPA make a variety of errors, such as deleting small grammatical terms, wrongly employing word ends and verb tenses, and/or messing up word order in phrases. Some people may eventually develop swallowing difficulties as well as more generalized motor symptoms, comparable to those found in movement-predominant FTDs such as corticobasal syndrome.

Signs and symptoms:

- Apraxia—difficulty making the necessary lip and tongue movements for speech. This causes distorted or inaccurate speech sounds, as well as slow, strained speech and groping facial and lip motions in an attempt to generate the correct sound. The initial symptom is generally labored speaking. Words with several syllables are the most difficult to create.

- Agrammatism—due to omissions and inaccuracies, speech becomes limited to short, simple phrases that are difficult to understand by the listener.

- Difficulty understanding long or grammatically difficult sentences. Single-word comprehension is unchanged, but the capacity to grasp long or grammatically difficult sentences is impaired. People with PPA may find it more difficult to comprehend what they see as "too much" verbal information, such as watching television or following a group conversation.

- Mutism

- Difficulty swallowing-This occurs later in the disease's course.

- Movement impairments similar to Parkinson's disease can arise. Slow, stiff movement, loss of balance or falling easily, trouble moving an arm or leg, and restricted up-and-down eye movement are all possible symptoms.

4.3 Logopenic variant of PPA

When speaking, people with logopenic variation PPA (lvPPA, also known as PPA-L) have trouble choosing words. As a result, individuals may speak slowly and pause frequently while searching for the appropriate word. They can still remember the meanings of words, unlike persons with semantic variant PPA. Speech can be absolutely fluent during the small discussion but become hesitant and halting when the person has to be particular or use a more unfamiliar word, unlike persons with agrammatic PPA. Speech is normally unforced and undistorted. The lvPPA type also has a short attention span for words, which makes it difficult to repeat phrases and sentences. As the condition advances, those who are affected may have difficulty understanding complex sentences.

Signs and symptoms:

- Impaired single-word retrieval

    - Finding the correct word while speaking is difficult.

    - Due to the time required for word recovery, there are pauses and hesitations.

    - An extended description (circumlocution) can be used to replace a lost word.

- **Impaired repetition**-Longer phrases and sentences pose more difficulty.

- **Phonological speech errors**-Omissions and substitutions in speech sounds are examples of mistakes. For instance, the affected individual may substitute sounds made at the tip of the tongue, such as "t" or "d," for sounds made near the neck, such as "k" or "g," as in "tup" instead of "cup" or "dap" instead of "gap." They can remove final consonants, such as "slee" rather than "sleep."

- **Phonological paraphasias**-A non-word with some of the same sounds is substituted for a real word. For example, the affected person might say "lelephone" instead of "telephone."

- Poor comprehension of complex sentences-With single-word comprehension spared.

- **Difficulty swallowing**-This may develop later in the progression of the disease.

5. Speech, language, and communication assessment of PPA

5.1 History

First, a thorough medical history is taken to determine whether a dementia condition, as stated above, exists. Because the patient may be ignorant of the symptoms (as in the case of memory loss or personality changes) or unable to describe them owing to aphasia, family members or friends are frequently questioned about the patient's behavior.

Case history and interview:

- It is critical that a thorough case history be obtained.
- Document the initial presentation as well as the emergence of any additional symptoms over time.
- Pay attention to characteristics of speech and language. At the time of evaluation, the degree of linguistic versus cognitive or motoric impairment (e.g., word-finding difficulties, agrammatism, phonological errors)
- Nonverbal cognitive deficits that could worsen over time (e.g., episodic memory impairment).
- Atypical behavioral symptoms (e.g., disinhibition, apathy, loss of empathy) that can arise, particularly in semantic variant PPA, or motoric symptomatology (e.g., limb apraxia, Parkinsonism, dysphagia) that can develop, most commonly in nonfluent/agrammatic PPA. If not previously indicated in the medical record, any family history of dementia or other pertinent medical diagnoses (particularly neurodegenerative disorders) should be investigated.
- Disabilities in hearing and/or vision should be documented.
- Whether the person is monolingual, bilingual, or multilingual.

  The therapist should enquire about existing functional communication demands and constraints in order to inform therapy planning. It's crucial, for example, to figure out which communication contexts (work, home, community), partners (family, friends, coworkers), and modes (telephone, face-to-face, written) are most significant in the patient's daily life. If possible, include the individual's primary communication partner(s) to establish a thorough and accurate case history.

5.2 Neurological examination

A neurological examination is performed to see if there is evidence of dementia on a simple mental function screening (the mental status assessment) as well as signs of motor or sensory symptoms that indicate various forms of neurological illnesses could be causing dementia. The neurologist may also arrange tests, such as an MRI scan, to rule out the possibility of a stroke or tumor as the cause of the symptoms.

5.3 Brain imaging studies

This can be done with a CAT scan or an MRI scan. Both of these technologies create an image of the brain, allowing any structural abnormalities like a stroke, tumor, or hydrocephalus—all of which can cause dementia-like symptoms—to be recognized.

The CAT scan and MRI scans in the case of degenerative brain disease may reveal "atrophy," which indicates "shrinkage" of the brain tissue, or they may not show anything at all, especially in the early stages. In fact, the report is frequently returned as "normal." However, this just implies that no evidence of a tumor or stroke exists. It is unable to provide information on the microscopic degenerative changes that have occurred.

5.4 Neuropsychological examination

It provides a more thorough assessment of mental health. This is especially crucial in the early stages of sickness, when a standard screening examination may fail to discover the patient's difficulties. This takes several hours and consists of tests of mental talents, such as attention and focus, language learning and memory, visual perception, logic, and mood, conducted by paper and pencil or computer. The results can reveal whether there are any irregularities in thought or behavior, as well as their severity (mild, moderate, or severe). Because we normally test memory by telling someone something and then asking them to repeat it later, demonstrating that people with PPA have intact memory can be difficult. In an individual with PPA, it may be impossible to repeat back the information because of the aphasia.

As a result, it's critical that testing is done adequately to ensure that there is not an actual memory loss. To yet, the only way to objectively diagnose dementia is to undergo a neuropsychological evaluation. There are currently no dementia-specific blood tests or other physiological diagnostics available. This is especially helpful if the symptoms are modest or in the early stages.

5.5 Psychiatric evaluation

Sometimes there will also be a need for a psychiatric evaluation. This may be the case when it is not clear if the changes in behavior are due to depression or another psychiatric disturbance.

5.6 Physiological evaluation

PPA impacts not just the person who is afflicted with the disorder, but also those who are close to them. Relationships, the ability to continue working, the ability to execute numerous ordinary tasks, and the ability to convey even the most basic requirements are all affected by the disease. Although there are several resources accessible for people with memory loss, there are far fewer resources available for people with PPA, their relatives, and friends. A consultation with a social professional who is experienced with PPA can address these concerns and offer advice on how to deal with daily frustrations and problems.

5.7 Speech and language evaluation

Because the primary symptom of PPA is a reduction in language abilities, it's critical to figure out which aspects of language use are most affected, how badly they are affected, and what may be done to improve communication. A speech-language pathologist (SLP) examines various areas of language in-depth and might provide recommendations to improve communication. Family members should be included in treatment sessions to learn how to communicate more effectively.

5.8 Formal assessment

The following tests can be used to assess various functions in patients with PPA:

- Mini-Mental State Examination [11]
- The Graded Naming Test [12]
- Wechsler Memory Scale—Revised [13]
- Rey–Osterrieth Complex Figure [14]
- The Visual Object and Space Perception [15]
- The Pyramids and Palm Trees Test [16]

In the **Indian context**, the following tests prove to be valid:

- The Western Aphasia Battery would help to classify the extent and type of Aphasia in these patients but supplementary tests need to be used.
- Neuropsychological tests also help in arriving at a diagnosis.
- Model-based tests e.g., Psycholinguistic Assessments of Language Processing in Aphasia (PALPA) provide information on underlying 'processing' deficits.

5.9 Informal assessment

5.9.1 Assessment of cognitive and linguistic functions:

1. Semantic memory:
    - Recognition of familiar faces.
    - Draw or color objects from memory, classify photographs using semantic criteria or match pictures of objects based on semantic similarity.
    - Executive functions, verbal fluency, and behavior: Impaired verbal fluency is frequently associated with executive function deficits such as abstraction (interpretation of proverbs, cognitive estimates, explaining similarities and differences), response inhibition, or motor sequencing (e.g. alternating hand movements).
    - The ability to create a list of common animals ("category fluency") or words beginning with a nominated letter ("phonological" or "phonemic fluency") can be used to measure verbal fluency.

- Progressive Nonfluent Aphasia (PNFA) is indicated by decreased letter fluency.
- The amount of words produced in one minute is used to determine the score.

2. Spontaneous speech:
    - The patient can be asked to describe a scene in a photograph or drawing, and the system will analyze an extended sample of the patient's spontaneous (propositional) speech.
    - This is preferable to asking the patient to describe a typical day in their life.

- Observing the patient's overall demeanor and demeanor during the clinical interview.
- Frontal dementia is a type of dementia that affects people in a passive way.
- PNFA is a group of people who are frustrated by their issues and try to compensate by using a lot of nonverbal gestures.
- Semantic dementia is characterized by a constant stream of circumlocutory speech.

3. Naming:
   - Naming should be assessed both in response to pictorial items (confrontational naming) and in response to verbal descriptions (e.g., "a large grey animal with a trunk").
   - The performance of naming should be evaluated for both high and low-frequency words (e.g., "shoe" versus "moat").
   - Examine if phonological (initial letter) or semantic (related item) cueing improves performance.
   - On confrontational naming tasks, visual perception deficits emerge as "visual" errors.
   - Circumlocutory reactions, semantic and phonological paraphasias can be noted.
   - Cueing with the first letter of the target word may help people with primary word retrieval and phonological encoding impairments (rather than primary verbal store faults).
   - Personal names might be particularly challenging.
4. Speech comprehension:
   - Word-finding and language output difficulties coexist.
   - Can be measured at the level of individual words, which is dependent on both intact perceptual systems and the verbal knowledge store (vocabulary), and sentences, which is dependent on the ability to maintain verbal information online and understand grammatical relationships between words.
5. Single-word comprehension:
   - Can be proven at the bedside by testing phoneme pair discrimination (for example, "pat—tap," and "gat—cat").
   - Noun comprehension—asking the patient to point to items mentioned or described by the examiner, to provide a definition or other information regarding a target word (e.g., "What is a squirrel?"), or to choose between possible synonyms for a target word (e.g., does "trench" mean "hedge" or "ditch"?).

- Asking the patient to classify items according to predetermined criteria (for example, "Is a lion a mammal?") can be used to dig further.

- When more fine-grained classifications are impossible, meaning is usually kept for broad categories of nouns.

- Comprehension of verbs can also be tested by having the patient choose an appropriate description of the examiner's actions ("pushing" versus "pulling", "catching" versus "throwing," etc.) or by asking them to do acts suggested by the examiner.

- Gestures can also be utilized as an assessment technique.

6. Sentence comprehension:

- A short sequence of acts following unique grammatical norms (e.g., "put the paper beneath the pen that is on the book," "you take up the watch, then give me the book") could be used to examine this.

- The patient could also be asked to recognize an image based on a syntactical sentence description (for example, "point to the boy being chased by the dog").

- Grammar comprehension can be separated into two types: syntactical (word relationships) and morphological (word changes in response to grammatical context), each with its own neurological foundations.

- You can test this by having the patient look for grammatical errors in written sentences.

- An early selective deficit in comprehending grammatical relations may be found in PNFA whereas in SD, comprehension of syntactical constructions is typically intact within the limitations of reduced vocabulary.

7. Speech repetition:

- Patients with impaired speech processing (such as word deafness) as well as those with impaired speech output are at risk.

- It's possible to assess it at the word and sentence level.

- Single-word repetition is frequently preserved in SD, although sentence repetition is influenced by understanding level.

- When individual words are lost, phonemes may "migrate" between words (for example, "the flag was colored bright red" may become "the blag was fullered with a right breg"), implying that the utterance is encoded as an extended sequence of phonemes (and thus susceptible to re-ordering), rather than a series of meaningful units).

8. Reading, writing, and spelling:

- The patient should be asked to read a piece aloud that contains both irregular and non-words (e.g. proper nouns).

- When reading a passage aloud, the sorts of errors produced convey information about the underlying reading fault.

- Rather than a core language impairment, patients who demonstrate letter-by-letter reading have a problem processing visual word forms: a syndrome of higher-order visual perception (the input to the verbal lexicon).

- Patients with verbal knowledge store deficits (in particular, SD) frequently "regularize" irregular words (e.g., reading "yacht" as "yatched"): this is a "surface dyslexia" [15, 17], in which reading is based on superficial rules for translating written words to speech sounds, rather than a learned vocabulary that governs the pronunciation.

- Regularization issues are particularly obvious for lower-frequency phrases.

- The loss of spelling vocabulary is a defining feature of the SD condition. Despite appropriate noun rendering, phonological dysgraphia (impaired spelling by sound) produces difficulties writing grammatical function words and non-words in PNFA [18].

- Written expression is often better retained with fewer errors than speech in patients with primary speech production impairments (for example, early in the course of PNFA).

9. Sentence generation and completion:

    - Once other linguistic functions have been established, this level can be judged with confidence.

    - Tasks that demand the development of novel verbal thought, such as the production of a statement including a target word (e.g. "boat") or the completion of an unfinished phrase, can be used to test the deficiency.

10. Motor assessment:

    - It is helpful to distinguish these from any linguistic loss, as well as to progress the clinical diagnosis in general.

    - The patient can be instructed to repeat a single syllable quickly (for example, "pa, pa, pa...") [19, 20]

    - Dysarthric patients' performance will be wrong if their rate or rhythm varies, although AOS patients' performance is normally normal.

    - AOS has a higher rate of sequencing mistakes.

5.9.2 Assessments designed for differential diagnosis and tracking severity in PPA

- Nine neuropsychological evaluations were created or altered expressly for the diagnosis or characterization of PPA, according to a recent systematic review. Several of these can be used to distinguish between clinical variations, and two of them were created expressly to assess PPA severity and progression.

- The Sydney Language Battery (SydBat) is a short battery of tests (image naming, word comprehension, semantic association, and repetition) that can be used to distinguish between PPA subtypes (80% accuracy).

- The Repeat and Point Test requires patients to repeat 10 multisyllabic words and point to the goal among semantic and phonological distractors in order to distinguish between semantic and nonfluent versions (100% accuracy).

- The Progressive Aphasia Severity Scale (PASS) is a tool used to assess symptoms and follow progression in people with PPA. On a three-point scale, clinicians rate the severity of speech and language deficits (articulation, fluency, syntax/grammar, word retrieval/expression, repetition, auditory comprehension phrases/sentences, single-word comprehension, reading, writing, and functional communication) as well as pragmatic aspects of communication. After an informant fills out a questionnaire and a structured interview with both the patient and the informant, the SLP completes the scale. **Table 1** describes PASS.

- The Progressive Aphasia Language Scale (PALS) includes clinician ratings of speech-language features (motor speech and grammatical features in spontaneous speech, naming, single word repetition and comprehension, and sentence repetition and comprehension), but it is based on signs observed during a prescribed set of speech-language tasks rather than symptoms reported via interview or questionnaire. PPA participants were subtyped by variation using an algorithm based on four essential aspects from this evaluation (motor speech impairment, grammar, single-word comprehension, and sentence repetition) (relative to expert clinical diagnosis).

- Clinical Dementia Rating (CDR), a dementia severity rating scale based on a semi-structured interview and clinical judgment, now includes a language domain, which improves sensitivity (relative to the original CDR) for detecting and tracking symptoms and functional impairments in language-prominent dementias like PPA.

5.9.3 Quality of life assessment

1. Communication Activities of Daily Living—3rd edition (CADL-3)

2. Assessment for Living with Aphasia (ALA)

3. Quality of Communication Life Scale (ASHA QCL)

4. American Speech-Language-Hearing Association Functional Assessment of Communication Skills for Adults (ASHA FACS)

5.10 Probable intervention strategies

5.10.1 Care, support, and treatment team of PPA

1. Neurologist (specialists in brain disorders who make the diagnosis and monitors its symptoms)

2. Neuropsychologist (evaluate cognitive abilities through specialized paper and pencil tests).

3. Psychiatrist (assist with behavioral and mood symptoms).

4. Social worker (help families navigate the difficult decisions related to their diagnosis).

PASS Domain	0 = Normal	0.5 = Questionable or very mild impairment	1 = Mild impairment	2 = Moderate impairment	3 = Sever impairment
FLUENCY-Degree to which speech flows easily, or it is interrupted by hesitations, pauses, fillers; reduced fluency is accompanied by decreased phrase length and words per minute.	Normal flow of speech	Speech contains occasional blank pauses or use fillers; reduced WPM and/or phrase length	Speech is in short phrases interrupted by pauses or groping for words but it is occasional	Dysfluencies in most utterances; phrase length rarely exceeds three words.	Severely dysfluent speech, phrase length rarely exceeds one word. May not speak.
SYNTAX AND GRAMMAR: Use of word forms, function words, and word order when forming phrases and sentences in most used modality (speech or writing)	No difficulty in the use of grammar and syntax	Occasional agrammatism or pragmatism (i.e odd sentence structure such as "I my car drive in your house') may complain it is effortful to combine words into phrases or sentences	Frequent agrammatism; sentence structures are simple; frequent misuse or omission of grammatical words or sentences	Utterances contain mostly content words with rare use of syntactic words, grouping; functional words or morphological markers	Single word utterances or no speech or writing.
SINGLE WORD COMPREHENSION: Ability to understand spoken or written a single word.	No difficulty in an understanding a single word in conversation or text.	Occasional difficulty in understanding, low-frequency words (eg: cork); may question the meaning of words (what?...)	Display lack of word comprehension several times in a brief conversation but able to carry out an easy reasonable meaningful conversation.	Understands some high frequency and / familiar words. Questions the meaning of many words in conversation.	Minimal comprehension of single word comprehension.

Table 1.
Three representative domains of the progressive aphasia severity scale (PASS) [21].

5. Speech and language pathologist (provide strategies to maximize communication abilities).

6. Physical and occupational therapists (help optimize movement and activities of daily living).

The goal is effective communication, not perfection as PPA is a progressive disorder. Early treatment, a specific plan, partner training, and long-term planning are all critical aspects of proper speech therapy treatment. Speech-language pathologists are uniquely competent to assess the present impact on communication, establish patient priorities, and build a treatment plan based on compensatory methods with a home program to preserve abilities as long as possible. We cannot stop PPA from progressing, but speech-language pathologists can help clients and families adjust their lives, compensate for their impairments, and keep the highest function and quality of life possible.

5.10.2 Tips for treating primary progressive aphasia

5.10.2.1 Practice priority vocabulary

- Practice only what is important to your client.
- Carryover does not occur.
- Create opportunities for your client to practice important words and phrases.
- Use of strategies like "cue cards".

5.10.2.2 Teach scripts for primary progressive aphasia

- If the client's main progressive aphasia is still in its early stages, have the family and the client pay attention to everyday routines and words. Request that a family member jots down your ideas. You'll now have a list of what's significant in the client's daily life, and you can use these phrases as scripts to practice as the PPA progresses.
- Speaking scripts can be used for a variety of situations, including:
  A typical discussions.
- Making a restaurant reservation.
- Calls that are made on a regular basis.
- Written scripts/models can be used for the following:
- Email
- Texts
- Check-writing
- Guidelines for writing effective scripts:

Depending on the severity of the PPA, vary the number and complexity of the scripts—the fewer and simpler the scripts, the more severe the PPA. Concentrate on clarity and reduce frustration. When in doubt, keep the script simple—you are not trying to teach something new; instead, you are bolstering and compensating. Set priorities based on the client's priorities.

5.10.2.3 Train compensatory strategies for primary progressive aphasia

Identifying and applying communication strengths can help you decide successful compensating measures and increase confidence, just as it can with aphasia or dementia. Modify hobbies and activities so that the person can compensate for linguistic difficulties. Labeling items in the environment is sometimes all that is required.

Clients should practice employing techniques, alternative communication, and scripts with the SLP, their family, and close friends in comfortable contexts. It will be easier to use them in public as a result of this.

5.10.2.4 Create a PPA business card

Individualized information cards may be beneficial to clients who are still self-sufficient in the community. This card can be used to inform people that the individual has aphasia, as well as what tactics can help and who to contact in an emergency. This can come in handy if the individual is having trouble at the grocery store or library, or if they have a run-in with the cops. Cards can also be used as a script for ordering a cup of coffee or checking in for tea time.

- To make contacts with new communication partners easier, hand out a customized card that describes what PPA is.

- Make sure the card is in a familiar position for the client, such as their pocketbook or purse, adjacent to their driver's license or photo ID. The card should include any relevant information that the person feels comfortable revealing, such as:

    - Name

    - Explanation of the communication difficulty or diagnosis (consider including that they are not drunk or on drugs, as is often assumed)

    - Quick communication tip strategy that can help (e.g. "use short phrases", "speak slowly", "allow extra time to understand", "be patient").

    - Emergency contact person's name and phone number.

5.10.2.5 Train nonverbal communication

Nonverbal skills become even more critical as PPA advances and communication abilities (especially verbal skills) deteriorate. Nonverbal communication is frequently easier to comprehend and produce. Teach care partners how to use gestures, eye contact, and body language and how to pay attention to them. Allow for more thinking time, have them write keywords, use visuals (photos, drawings, objects), shorten their phrases, and so on.

5.10.2.6 Voice banking and AAC

When words fail, care partners can use AAC apps to help communicate their message. Early on in therapy, you can try out different AAC apps to discover which one or style the client enjoys, and then start customizing and training them before they are needed.

5.10.2.7 Plan for the future

From the first day of treatment, the focus should be on a home program and compensating methods. Set up routines and experiment with multimodal and alternative communication as soon as possible, even before the client requires it. It will be easier to understand and acquire new strategies and routines early in the disease process, while more language and cognitive skills are still intact. Clients and families have more time to become comfortable with communication options and select what they like and do not like with earlier involvement. If at all possible, follow up with the client after discharge or check in with them every few months. PPA's home program and communication tactics will need to evolve as his or her life progresses.

5.10.3 Phased treatment

Clinicians need to consider important differences when managing speech and language impairments in the context of progressive disease [22].

In aphasia caused by stroke, clients show a static or gradually improving communication profile. But clients with PPA will eventually become mute or speak largely in jargon—using words that have some meaning to them but not to the listener.

Ultimately, with the disease's progression, patients will show increasing cognitive, behavioral, and motor deterioration.

Given this trajectory, PPA treatment should address a client's current profile of spared and impaired abilities, while also addressing the client's inevitable decline in communication and, in later stages, other domains.

Because of the evolving nature of PPA, a phased treatment approach, with recurring assessment and repeated treatment "doses" tailored to the client's current communication needs and challenges is recommended.

5.10.3.1 Phase 1—restitutive treatment in mild PPA

- A crucial part of the SLP's role during the early stages of PPA is to thoroughly evaluate and document the patient's communication. This initial evaluation serves as the baseline for the progression of difficulties and helps to identify targets for treatment.

- Clinician often focuses on rebuilding impaired communicative abilities via recitative treatments.

- Treatment during mild stages is critical for helping clients relearn lost skills.

5.10.3.2 Phase 2—toward aided communication in moderate PPA

- Treatment shifts toward multimodal communication and the use of augmentative and alternative communication (AAC).

- Select functional phrases and words to include.

- Strategies to maximize conversational success.

- Also provides counseling regarding PPA.

5.10.3.3 Phase 3—environmental support and communication partner training in moderate-severe to severe PPA

- Treatment focuses on communication partner training and environmental modifications.

- This phased treatment approach allows clinicians to draw from their experience treating aphasia while taking into account the inevitable decline associated with PPA.

5.10.4 Promoting self-cueing strategies

SLPs should focus on self-cueing strategies for lexical retrieval in the mild phases of PPA, which take advantage of the individual's residual skills [4]. During the examination, semantic, orthographic, and phonological self-cueing should all be tested in order to discover which method is most effective in prompting retrieval.

Family members can be taught to use cueing tactics like "Tell me about it" or "Can you think of what letter it starts with?" to help initiate self-cueing. The ultimate goal is for the person to be able to self-cue at the conversational level on their own. The SLP must be aware, however, when the family member is working too hard or seeing all interactions in therapy sessions.

5.10.5 Script training

Researchers have shown that conversational scripts can help people with stroke-induced aphasia improving their functional communication [23, 24]. The advantage of script training is the automaticity with which patients acquire skills by recalling memories of context-bound, skilled performance. When the same stimuli from the practice environment are available in a functional context, repeated practice of a specific task might improve automatic retrieval. The key to script training is to make sure that each person practices consistently and thoroughly. The SLP should consider the individual's requirements and interests, the style of the script (dialog or monolog), the number and duration of conversational turns, as well as the grammatical complexity and vocabulary choices when writing a script [25]. Families may purchase a script computer program such as Aphasia Scripts.

Examples of possible script topics include:

- Talking to a family member or friend (e.g. by phone).

- Scheduling an appointment; asking for directions.

- Stating personal information or explaining PPA.

- Giving a lecture or speech

- Saying prayers.

SLPs can frame a written goals based on the accuracy and rate of production (e.g., timing how long it takes to read the script while counting the number of errors). If the person is not motivated to practice the script outside of therapy sessions, he or she may not be a good candidate for script training.

5.10.6 Facilitating receptive language

Facilitating the use of Receptive Language Family training on ways to aid comprehension is critical for individuals with receptive language difficulties. Automatically speaking communication partners can make a difference in comprehension.

- Talk softly, face the person, and give them your undivided attention.
- Augmenting speech with motions.
- Only giving one command at a time.
- Employing grammatical structures and terminology that are easy to understand, or.
- Removing distractions from crucial conversations (e.g., turning off the TV/radio).

5.10.7 Low-tech AAC

The SLP's job is to determine the book's proper format, font size, and word/page length, and then instruct the individual and family members to keep adding pages.

- When creating a communication book, SLPs should think about a few things.
- SLPs can laminate small photographs so that the patient can attach them to a key ring and carry them in his or her pocket.
- SLPs should utilize plastic page protectors in a binder to create a more thorough book.
- Using images from the Internet or the person's own photographs, SLPs can personalize pages.
- SLPs can break the book into sections using tabs.
- SLPs should ask family members to record words and ideas that have led to communication breakdowns. They should add these to the book.

Because some individuals with PPA may not independently use the book, training the family members on appropriate cueing strategies to initiate book use and facilitate navigation also should be targeted during treatment sessions.

5.10.8 High-tech AAC devices

Despite the lack of evidence on AAC intervention options for people with PPA, SLPs have effectively used high-tech AAC devices to help people with severe aphasia caused by stroke communicate [26]. Because people with PPA's other cognitive abilities deteriorate with time, it's crucial to keep in mind that a person's capacity to learn to utilize high-tech equipment may be limited and eventually hampered. The SLP's job is to figure out which devices if any, will best enable the client to convey his or her needs and allow for social communication. The SLP should ask a series of questions to determine if a high-tech AAC is a good fit for someone with PPA.

- Is the person enthusiastic about using a high-tech ACC to communicate? Otherwise, it is unlikely to succeed.
- Can the person operate other types of technology independently, such as a computer, microwave, TV remote, or phone? If not, this could suggest a loss of fine motor skills or an inability to sequence, indicating that you are not a good candidate for an ACC.
- Has the family member(s) been involved in the planning, training, and achievement of the objectives? If not, invite family members to several sessions to ensure that the plan is implemented successfully.
- Has the person and their family been taught how to utilize the device in everyday situations? Have the trials attained their objectives? If not, consider additional training and a long trial.
- In conclusion, people with PPA have a variety of choices for increasing communication. Patients and their families are advised to follow the following guidelines:
- In the early stages of the disease, a comprehensive evaluation of speech, language, and other cognitive abilities should be sought.
- Follow-up evaluations are required on a regular basis to evaluate patterns of language deterioration.
- Treatment should begin as soon as possible, focusing on the areas of speech and language that are affected.
- As language abilities deteriorate, the treatment focus should be modified.
- Early on, augmentative communication strategies should be implemented. Patients who are given these tactics later in their language loss may find it difficult to learn how to use them.
- Involving family members or other people with whom the patient talks are critical not just for increasing awareness of effective communication tactics, but also for practicing them with the patient.
- As patients' ability to communicate fades, they will rely increasingly on augmentative communication tools. With individual patients, some techniques may be more effective than others, and some patients may utilize more than one.
- Treatment will not stop the aphasia from progressing, but it will considerably improve communication abilities.

6. General suggestions for communicating with individuals with PPA

*Communication is usually most successful in a peaceful, calm, relaxed situation. Avoid talks when the television is on, and avoid circumstances where numerous individuals are talking at the same time. Avoiding social circumstances is not necessary; rather, such activities should be encouraged. Maintain usual activities as much as feasible. When people are not tired, communication is usually the most effective.

Communication partner	Individual with PPA
Be patient—give your partner time to communicate.	Remember, your partner is trying, so be patient.
The main goal is the communication of information—not speech or perfection. Once information has been communicated, move on.	The main goal is to communicate—not speech or perfection. Use whatever methods you can to get your message across—speech, writing, drawing, gesture and/or communication notebook. Ask for help when needed.
Be careful not to speak too quickly.	Take your time.
Ask questions one at a time, pausing between each. Ask yes/no questions, or multiple choice questions.	Try to give as much relevant information as possible. Focus on expressing the "main points."
Repeat what you understand to clarify.	Ask your partner to repeat if you do not understand what was said. Use facial expressions to indicate when you misunderstand.
Treat the individual as an adult. Do not talk down. Intelligence is generally intact; communication is the problem.	

Author details

Yashaswini Channabasave Gowda[1] and Hema Nagaraj[2*]

1 Junior Research Fellow, Department of Speech-Language Sciences, All India Institute of Speech and Hearing, Mysore, India

2 Assistant Professor, Department of Speech-Language Sciences, All India Institute of Speech and Hearing, Mysore, India

*Address all correspondence to: hema_chari2@yahoo.com

References

[1] Ferrano A, Jervis GA. Pick's disease. Archives of Neurology and Psychiatry. 1936;**36**:739-767

[2] Weintraub S, Rubin NP, Mesulam MM. Primary progressive aphasia: Longitudinal course, neuropsychological profile, and language features. Archives of Neurology. 1990;**47**(12):1329-1335

[3] Pick A. der linksseitigen Schläfenlappenatrophie. Monatsschrift für Psychiatrie und Neurologie. 1904;**16**:378

[4] Löwenberg K. Pick's disease: A clinicopathologic contribution. Archives of Neurology and Psychiatry. 1936;**36**(4):768-789

[5] Mesulam MM, Weintraub S. Primary progressive aphasia: Sharpening the focus on a clinical syndrome. In: Heterogeneity of Alzheimer's Disease. Berlin, Heidelberg: Springer; 1992. pp. 43-66

[6] Warrington EK. The selective impairment of semantic memory. The Quarterly Journal of Experimental Psychology. 1975;**27**(4):635-657

[7] Schwartz MF, Marin OS, Saffran EM. Dissociations of language function in dementia: A case study. Brain and Language. 1979;**7**(3):277-306

[8] Duffy JR, Petersen RC. Primary progressive aphasia. Aphasiology. 1992;**6**(1):1-15

[9] Martin A. Neuropsychology of Alzheimer's disease: The case for subgroups Alex Martin. Modular Deficits in Alzheimer-type Dementia. 1990;**143**:a006171

[10] Mesulam MM. Primary progressive aphasia. Annals of Neurology. 2001;**49**(4):425-432

[11] Folstein MF, Folstein SE, McHugh PR. "Mini-mental state": A practical method for grading the cognitive state of patients for the clinician. Journal of Psychiatric Research. 1975;**12**(3):189-198

[12] Mckenna P, Warrington EK. Graded Naming Test: Manual. UK: NFERNelson; 1983

[13] Wechsler D. Wechsler Memory Scale-Revised. Berlin: Psychological Corporation; 1987

[14] Rey A. L'examen clinique en psychologie. Paris: Presses Universitaires de France; 1964

[15] Warrington EK, James M. Visual object recognition in patients with right-hemisphere lesions: Axes or features? Perception. 1986;**15**(3):355-366

[16] Howard D, Patterson K. The pyramids and palm trees test. In: A Test of Semantic Access from Words and Pictures. Bury St. Edmunds: Thames Valley Company; 1992

[17] Marshall JC, Newcombe F. Patterns of paralexia: A psycholinguistic approach. Journal of Psycholinguistic Research. 1973;**2**(3):175-199

[18] Graham NL, Patterson K, Hodges JR. The impact of semantic memory impairment on spelling: Evidence from semantic dementia. Neuropsychologia. 2000;**38**(2):143-163

[19] Dabul B. Apraxia Battery for Adults. Austin, Texas: Pro-Ed; 2000

[20] Duffy JR, Strand EA, Josephs KA. Motor speech disorders associated with primary progressive aphasia. Aphasiology. 2014;**28**(8-9):1004-1017

[21] Sapolsky D, Bakkour A, Negreira A, Nalipinski P, Weintraub S,

Mesulam MM, et al. Cortical neuroanatomic correlates of symptom severity in primary progressive aphasia. Neurology. 2010;**75**:358-366. DOI: 10.1212/WNL.0b013e3181ea15e8

[22] Hinshelwood H, Henry M, Fromm D. Helping them hold on: Through phased treatment, speechlanguage pathologists can help clients with primary progressive aphasia function as normally as possible—For as long as they can. The ASHA Leader. 2016;**21**(10):44-51

[23] Youmans G, Holland A, Muñoz M, Bourgeois M. Script training and automaticity in two individuals with aphasia. Aphasiology. 2005;**19**(3-5):435-450

[24] Youmans G, Youmans SR, Hancock AB. Script training treatment for adults with apraxia of speech. American Journal of Speech-Language Patholog. 2011;**20**:23-27

[25] Cherney LR, Halper AS, Kaye RC. Computer-based script training for aphasia: Emerging themes from posttreatment interviews. Journal of Communication Disorders. 2011;**44**(4):493-501

[26] Beukelman DR, Fager S, Ball L, Dietz A. AAC for adults with acquired neurological conditions: A review. Augmentative and Alternative Communication. 2007;**23**(3):230-242

Section 2

The Outcome and Treatment of Aphasias

Chapter 5

Spontaneous Recovery and Intervention in Aphasia

Chiaki Yamaji and Shinichiro Maeshima

Abstract

The recovery of aphasia occurs immediately after the onset of the disease and lasts for several months or more. The speed and degree of improvement in aphasia vary depending on the time since onset, severity of aphasia, and each language modalities. It is assumed that there is a difference in the mechanism of aphasia recovery. The recovery process of the central nervous system observed in the first few days to weeks after the onset of aphasia is thought to involve the disappearance of cerebral edema, the absorption of necrotic tissue, angiogenesis, the development of the collateral circulation, and the resolution of hematomas, leading to the repair of damaged tissue. In the chronic phase, 1) recovery of damaged functional areas, 2) reconstruction of functions in the residual areas, and 3) compensatory functions by the contralateral hemisphere or activation of the contralateral cortex are assumed. In recent years, there have been many reports supporting the effectiveness of speech and language therapy interventions. Speech and language therapy should not only promote improvement of aphasia, but also take a comprehensive approach to improve the QOL of aphasia patients, such as acquisition of compensatory means of communication and family guidance.

Keywords: aphasia, spontaneous recovery, recovery process, speech language therapy, rehabilitation

1. Introduction

1.1 What is spontaneous recovery?

Spontaneous recovery from aphasia implies that impaired language functions improve without speech therapy interventions [1]. Several previous studies have investigated the duration for and degree of spontaneous recovery from aphasia. Culton evaluated the progress of improvement in language functions over a 2-month period four times at 2-week intervals using eight types of language tasks, such as naming and writing, in 11 patients with acute aphasia 2–4 weeks after the onset and in patients with chronic aphasia 11–48 months after the onset. Language therapy was not performed during the assessment period in both the groups. It has been reported that the acute aphasia group showed a more marked improvement. Particularly, the largest differences in the results of the language tasks were observed between the first and the second sessions, which indicated that the degree of improvement was most pronounced about 1 month following the onset of aphasia. It was also reported that improvements continued up to approximately 3 months after the onset [1]. Hartman (1981) evaluated language functions at the first visit and 30 days after the onset using the Porch Index of Communicative Ability (PICA) in 44 patients with acute aphasia within 2 weeks after the onset. Comparison was made between the early group, which consisted of 20 patients who were administered the PICA within 6 days after the onset, and the late group, which consisted of 24 patients who were administered the PICA 7–14 days after the onset. Speech therapy was not administered in either of the two groups. As 42 of 44 patients showed improvements, it was reported that spontaneous recovery was achieved within 1 month. In particular, the early group showed more improvement in scores, showing most pronounced spontaneous recovery within 1–2 weeks. Moreover, given that the results of the final PICA were positively correlated with those of the initial PICA, it was argued that the degree of spontaneous recovery might be proportional to the severity of aphasia at the time of the onset [2]. Lomas & Kertesz evaluated language functions within 30 days and 3 months after the aphasia onset using the Western Aphasia Battery (WAB) in 31 patients with poststroke aphasia. Based on the initial WAB results, the patients were divided into the following four groups: the non-fluent/poor comprehension group, non-fluent/good comprehension group, fluent/poor comprehension group, and fluent/good the comprehension group. The two good comprehension groups exhibited improvements in general language functions, whereas the two poor comprehension groups displayed great improvements in comprehension and repetition [3]. Maeshima et al. evaluated language functions 1, 3, and 6 months after the aphasia onset using the Standard Language Test of Aphasia (SLTA) in 30 patients with poststroke aphasia who had not received speech therapy. Regardless of the age and gender, the SLTA scores improved 3 months after the onset in 18 patients; particularly marked improvements were noted in patients with moderate/mild aphasia. The SLTA scores improved 6 months after the onset in 14 patients irrespective of the severity. In terms of language tasks, such as writing, speech, and comprehension, improvements were observed in all tasks within 6 months. However, differences in the degree of improvement depending on the type and severity of aphasia were reported. Additionally, they reported that some patients were still followed 9–12 months later and that improvements were noted even in patients with severe aphasia [4]. Lendrem & Lincoln used PICA to evaluate 52 patients with poststroke aphasia who did not receive speech therapy 4, 10, 22, and 34 weeks after the onset. They reported that improvements in language functions continued until 34 weeks with the most pronounced improvement at 4–10 weeks. In particular, the results of the first PICA were correlated with the language functions after 6 months, suggesting that the degree of improvement is proportional to the severity of aphasia at the onset [5]. Sarno and Levita evaluated language functions using the Functional Communication Profile (FCP) in 28 patients with severe poststroke aphasia who did not receive speech therapy within 2 days, at 3 and 6 months after the onset. They reported that, as some subjects passed away, the number of the subjects decreased to 18 after 3 months and 14 after 6 months, and the improvements in the FCP were more pronounced at 3 months than 6 months after the onset [6].

Based on these reports, it is clear that spontaneous recovery from aphasia is possible in some cases. Age and gender do not seem to greatly affect the recovery. Although the degree of recovery differs depending on the severity of aphasia and language functions, improvements may be most pronounced 1–3 months after the onset and continue for 3–6 months or more.

1.2 Mechanism involved in recovery of the central nervous system

The recovery process of the central nervous system for a few weeks after the onset is believed to involve reduction of brain edema, necrotic tissue absorption, hematoma absorption, and formation of collateral circulation. Although recovery of the central nervous system is limited after a long duration since the onset, language functions may continue to improve gradually.

Regarding the correlation between the recovery of language functions and the central nervous system recovery, Saur et al. conducted a study using functional magnetic resonance imaging (fMRI). They reported the following processes in acute-phase middle cerebral artery (MCA) infarction: First, the activation of the remaining language-associated brain area is reduced, then activation occurs in the brain area related to language function improvement as well as in the surrounding area and the contralateral hemisphere, and finally normal activation ensues. Therefore, the reorganization of the central nervous system progresses in a stepwise manner [7].

Heiss et al., using positron emission tomography, investigated language functions 2 and 8 weeks after the onset in 23 patients with poststroke aphasia. In the group including patients with frontal lobe lesions and in that including patients with subcortical lesions, the right inferior frontal gyrus and the right superior temporal gyrus (STG) were activated at 2 weeks, and the left STG was activated at 8 weeks, showing considerable improvements in the language functions. Among patients with temporal lobe lesions, the left Broca's area and the supplementary motor area were activated at 2 weeks, and the bilateral precentral gyri and the right STG were activated at 8 weeks. However, the left STG did not activate, and improvements in the language functions were negligible. They reported that the recovery of language functions is preceded by compensation in the right hemisphere and that the preservation of the left STG is crucial for the reorganization of the neural network [8].

Mimura et al. performed single photon emission computed tomography (SPECT) to investigate the relationship between cerebral blood flow and language functions in patients with aphasia caused by left MCA lesions within 1 year and 7 years after the onset. They argued that increased blood flow in the left hemisphere was correlated with changes in language functions at 3–9 months and that functional recovery of the left hemisphere was essential for the improvement in language functions within 1 year. Changes in language functions after 7 years were correlated with increases in blood flow in the right hemisphere (especially in the frontal lobe and the thalamus). Functional compensation by the contralateral hemisphere may be involved in the long-term recovery of language functions [9].

These previous reports suggest that the mechanism of recovery involved in central nervous system reorganization may differ depending on the time from the onset. The mechanism for central nervous system recovery may possibly involve the recovery of damaged functional areas, reorganization of neurons in the remaining areas, or compensation by the contralateral hemisphere.

Pani et al. investigated the correlation between the right hemisphere and language functions in patients with chronic aphasia. They reported that fluency of speech was highly correlated with the volume of the middle temporal gyrus, precentral gyrus, and inferior frontal gyrus in the right hemisphere, as well as the volume of the fibers connecting the right and left supplementary motor areas. This may reflect a predisposition toward compensatory functions of the contralateral hemisphere [10].

2. Improvement in language functions

2.1 Factors related to improvement in language functions

2.1.1 Age

Many reports state that young people are more likely to show greater improvement in language functions than old people [11–14]. The underlying factor for this difference is believed to be the difference in the plasticity of the brain associated with age. Previous studies using fMRI revealed that the left inferior frontal gyrus was activated in young subjects during verbal fluency tasks. Conversely, old subjects showed activation of the right inferior/middle frontal gyrus and poorer scores. These findings imply age-dependent differences in brain physiology and functions [15].

However, many reports conclude that there are no age-dependent differences in terms of improvement in language functions [1, 5, 16–24]. Therefore, no consensus has been reached on this matter. It is unlikely that language functions are related exclusively to age; hence, other factors, such as etiological causes (post-traumatic aphasia is prevalent in young people) and types of aphasia (Broca's aphasia is prevalent in young people), may also be related to language functions. Therefore, age-dependent differences may not have been apparent in studies that controlled these conditions. While age is an important factor for improving language functions, one must pay attention to the interpretation of correlation.

2.1.2 Gender

There are gender differences in terms of recovery from aphasia, and some reports showed that women were more inclined to recover than men [25, 26]. These differences may be attributed to the gender differences in the functional composition of the brain. Kansaku & Kitazawa conducted a study using fMRI and reported apparent gender-based differences in the activity of the anterior and posterior speech areas in vocabulary and story comprehension tasks, respectively [27]. Likewise, Shaywitz et al. also conducted a study using fMRI in which activation was found to be biased in the left inferior frontal gyrus in men in phonologic tasks, whereas broad areas including bilateral inferior frontal gyrus were found to be activated in women [28]. These reports indicate that gender plays a role in activating the brain areas with respect to language function. However, many reports argued that gender was not a factor for improving language functions [14, 16, 17, 19–21, 29]. Therefore, no definite correlation between gender and improvement in language functions has been established. Besides, other factors may also be related to gender. For instance, women are more susceptible than men to subarachnoid hemorrhage, which is an etiological factor conducive to improvement in language functions.

2.1.3 Causative diseases

Improvements in language functions are greater in patients with traumatic injury and in patients with brain hemorrhage than those in patients with brain infarction, respectively [29, 30]. This is attributable to differences in the extent of damage to the parenchyma in the cortical/subcortical tissue in the brain. Compared with brain infarction cases, brain hemorrhage cases achieve greater improvements through the absorption of hematoma and reduction of edema. However, severe aphasia may persist following traumatic injury and brain hemorrhage. Accordingly, prognoses may differ depending on the severity of brain damage. In addition, because of the differences in indications for thrombolysis or thrombectomy, it is difficult to predict the recovery of language function based on etiology alone today.

2.1.4 Dominant hand

The dominant hand is closely related to the language-dominant hemisphere, and 96%, 85%, and 73% of right-handed, ambidextrous, and left-handed people, respectively, have the left hemisphere predominantly controlling language functions [31]. The incidence of aphasia caused by damage to the right hemisphere in non-right-handed people is believed to be 20–40% [32, 33]. As with right-handed people, most non-right-handed people develop aphasia triggered by damage to the left hemisphere. It has been reported that left-handed people develop aphasia more often than right-handed people [34, 35]. Smith reported that there were few left handers in patients with residual aphasia in the chronic phase [36].

These reports suggest that left-handed people are more susceptible to aphasia, but they tend to experience quick and larger improvements in language functions. The following are considered to be factors for good prognosis in left-handed patients with aphasia: A larger brain area responsible for language functions is conducive to restoring any remaining functions, and the presence of areas controlling language functions in both the hemispheres facilitates the activation of compensatory functions in the intact hemisphere [37, 38]. Meanwhile, some reports documented that left-handed patients with aphasia caused by damage to the left hemisphere had poor prognosis [39, 40]. Accordingly, there may be individual differences in the hemispheric dominance of language functions in non-right-handed people.

Among right-handed patients, some may have potential predispositions for left-handedness, such as a history of forced adjustment and familial factors. Information needs to be collected thoroughly in this regard.

2.1.5 Severity of aphasia at the onset

Many reports stated that the severity of aphasia at the onset affects prognosis [5, 11, 16, 17, 19–21, 23, 29, 41, 42]. All these reports argued that the language functions improve slowly and quickly in patients with severe and mild aphasia at the onset, respectively. As some reports indicate that the severity of aphasia is proportional to the severity of stroke, there is a possibility that the severity of brain damage also determines the severity and prognosis of aphasia.

Meanwhile, Lazar et al. reported that many patients with severe aphasia could still improve and that there were considerable variations in the degree of improvement in language functions and severity of aphasia 90 days after the onset. Therefore, they concluded that estimating prognosis based on the initial severity alone may be difficult [18]. Mohr et al. investigated language functions in three patients with global aphasia for 5 years and reported that improvements were observed in all the functions, except naming [43]. All reports indicated that language functions may improve even in patients with severe aphasia at the onset. They also suggested that the period required for improvement may differ depending on the patient.

2.1.6 Types of aphasia at the onset

While some reports state that types of aphasia affect the improvement in language functions, others indicated that there is no relationship between them [24]. Kertesz and McCabe reported that Broca's aphasia showed the largest improvement, followed by conduction aphasia. They stated that amnestic aphasia did not achieve large improvements because it was mild at the onset. Regarding long-term prognosis, patients with global aphasia showed poor prognosis, whereas patients with Broca's and Wernicke's aphasias exhibited moderately poor prognosis. Complete recovery was achieved in many patients with amnesic aphasia, conduction aphasia, and transcortical aphasia [29]. Demeurisse et al. investigated prognosis 6 months after aphasia onset in patients with three different types of aphasia: global, Broca's, and Wernicke's. They reported that patients in the global aphasia group exhibited poorer improvements than those in the other two aphasia groups [41]. Bakheit et al. classified 75 patients with aphasia into the following groups based on the WAB classification: Broca's, Wernicke's, global, amnesic, and conduction aphasia, and administered the WAB at the onset and 4, 8, 12, and 24 weeks after the onset. Consequently, the Broca's aphasia group showed greater improvements than all the other groups, with the greatest improvement from the time of onset to 4 weeks after the onset [44]. Kertetsz reported that the rate of recovery differed depending on the type of aphasia, and patients with Broca's aphasia achieved the greatest improvement [19]. All these studies commonly reported that patients with Broca's aphasia had good prognoses, whereas patients with global aphasia showed poor prognoses. However, it should be noted that although patients with amnesic and conduction aphasias who had good WAB scores at the time of admission appeared to achieve less improvements due to a ceiling effect, their final scores tended to be higher than those of patients with Broca's aphasia who were known to show better improvements.

In a review, Watila and Balarabe cited the location and size of lesions, types of aphasia, and severity as the most critical factors for determining the recovery from aphasia. They concluded that, as all these factors are related each other, it would be difficult to investigate the independent factors [20]. The type of aphasia is somewhat consistent with the severity (e.g., amnestic aphasia is mild and global aphasia is severe). The location of lesions for non-fluent aphasia is different from that for fluent aphasia (anterior or posterior to the boundary of the central sulcus). Therefore, differences in aphasia types may be a factor encompassing these differences.

2.1.7 Location and size of lesions

Watila & Balarabe [20] and Plowman et al. [21] cited the location and size of lesions as factors contributing to the improvement in language functions in patients with poststroke aphasia. Maeshima et al. [45] investigated hemorrhage volume and language functions in 92 patients with putaminal hemorrhage. Consequently, they discovered that repetition difficulty was developed when the hemorrhage volume exceeded 20 mL, and non-fluent aphasia occurred when it exceeded 40 mL. The aforementioned causes of aphasia affect prognosis. However, prognosis may also differ depending on the location and size of lesions in the cortex or subcortex.

Regarding the location of lesions, Marchina et al. emphasized the importance of the arcuate fasciculus, stating that the degree of damage to the arcuate fasciculus is correlated with the improvement in spontaneous speech and naming [46]. The size of lesions represents the degree of damage to the area responsible for controlling language functions itself in the cortex. In the subcortex, improvements in language functions may be poor, despite the lesions being small, when the arcuate fasciculus is damaged.

As discussed above, many studies investigated factors contributing to the recovery of language functions, and all the cited factors were observed to interact and intertwine with each other. Because conditions were not controlled in previous studies, it is not easy to compare each of the factors; thus, no definite theory has been formulated. As most previous studies included patients who underwent speech therapy, it was difficult to clarify whether this was also related to spontaneous recovery.

2.2 Effects of speech and language therapy interventions

One of the effects of speech and language therapy interventions is the improvement in language functions, which is better than the improvement achieved by spontaneous recovery. Nowadays, because speech therapy is provided worldwide to such patients, it is difficult to clearly distinguish between speech therapy-induced recovery and spontaneous recovery. To assess the efficacy of speech and language therapy, previous studies comparing trained and non-trained cases serve as good references.

There are few negative reports on the effectiveness of speech and language therapy. Lincoln et al. investigated changes in language functions in the speech therapy group and the no-therapy group 22 and 34 weeks after the onset. The results showed that language functions improved in both the groups and that no significant differences were observed in the degree of recovery between the two groups [47]. Levita compared improvements in language functions between the group that received speech therapy for 8 weeks and the no-therapy group in patients with aphasia 4–12 weeks after the onset. No differences were found between the two groups [48].

Many reports support the efficacy of speech and language therapy. Wertz et al. compared improvements in language functions in the following three groups: a group of patients who received speech therapy by speech therapists from the onset to week 12 and did not receive any therapy from week 12 to 24; a group of patients who received language practice by volunteers until week 12 and did not receive any practice from week 12 to 24; and a group of patients who did not receive any therapy until week 12 and received speech therapy by speech therapists from week 12 to 24. The results showed that, as of week 12, significant differences were observed between the groups that received language therapy by speech therapists until week 12 and the group that did not receive any language therapy until week 12 and that no significant differences were observed among all the groups at 24 weeks. They concluded that language therapy by speech therapists promotes improvements at the onset, and delayed interventions are still conducive to improvements [49].

Basso et al. investigated the factors affecting the improvement in the four language functions of speech, comprehension, reading, and writing, in the speech therapy group, which consisted of 162 patients who underwent speech therapy and the no-treatment group, which consisted of 119 patients who did not. In this study, although the duration from the onset to language function evaluation varied greatly, they compared the results of the language function evaluation for the first time and after 6 months, and reported that the implementation of language therapy was a factor responsible for improvements in all the language functions [24].

Maeshima et al. examined the language functions (writing, speech, and comprehension) in the speech therapy group, which consisted of 18 patients who received language therapy and the no-treatment group, which consisted of 18 patients who did not. They compared scores for each function and also compared the comprehensive language function scores calculated by summing each function scores between the two groups, 1, 3, and 6 months after the onset. No significant differences were observed in the language functions at 1 and 6 months after the onset between the two groups. However, many patients in the speech therapy group showed significant improvements at 3 months after the onset (**Figure 1**). Based on language function, many patients in the speech therapy group improved with regard to speech and writing at 3 months after the onset (**Figure 2**). These results indicate that improvements beyond spontaneous recovery may be achieved at an early stage following speech therapy interventions. In particular, it is easier to obtain the effects on the expressive aspect of language functions [50].

These reports suggest that early administration of speech therapy facilitates the recovery process beyond spontaneous recovery. The intervention effects may include improvements not only in passive language functions but also in active language functions that cannot be easily facilitated by daily voice–language communication.

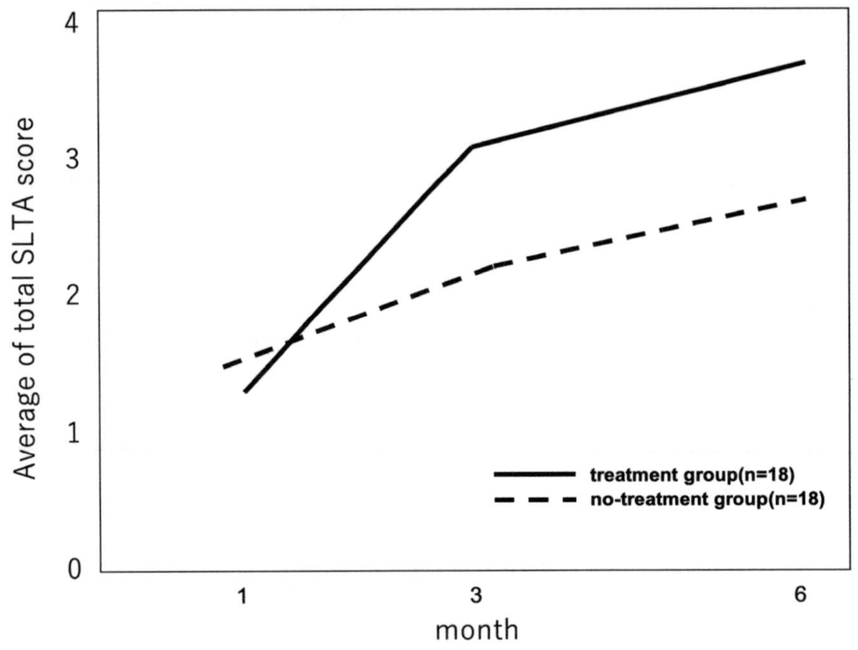

Figure 1.
Many patients in the speech therapy group showed significant improvements of language at 3 months after the onset.

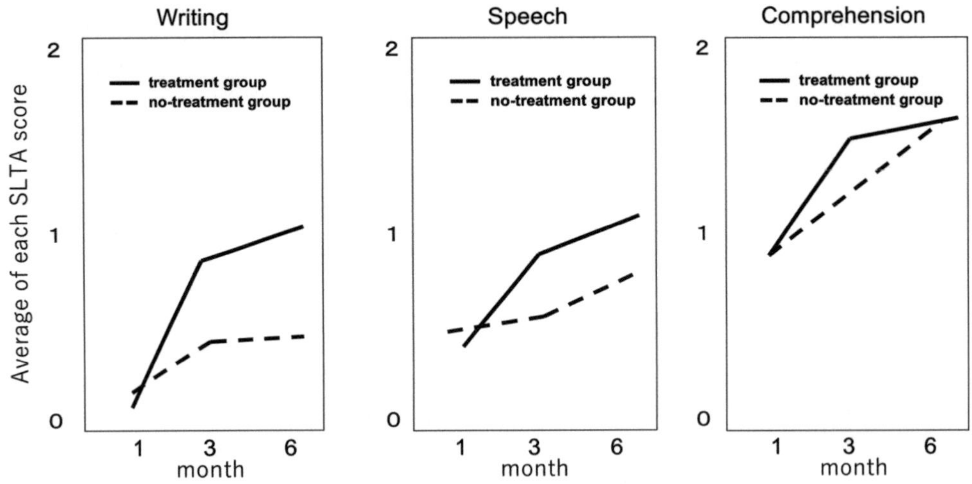

Figure 2.
Many patients in the speech therapy group improved with regard to speech and writing at 3 months after the onset.

In a literature review, Cicerone et al. stated that there was evidence supporting the efficacy of speech and language therapy for aphasia [51]. Conversely, while acknowledging the effectiveness of speech and language therapy, Mimura et al. argued in a review that scientific evidence was still insufficient because of the lack of evaluation of practice content's individuality and the effects in the no practice group [52]. In a Cochrane review, Brady et al. similarly stated that there was evidence supporting the effectiveness of speech therapy in improving functional communication, reading, writing, and expressive language, suggesting the efficacy of frequent and long-term speech therapy. However, they also argued that evidence was still insufficient because of small sample sizes and disunified practice methods [53]. Pickersgill and Lincoln (1983) asserted that although speech therapy interventions were expected to lead to early recovery, they would not expand the degree of final recovery. They appealed the early intervention effects of speech therapy, while simultaneously casting doubts regarding the argument that the interventions would also promote long-term recovery [23].

2.3 Significance of speech therapy interventions

As mentioned above, speech therapy interventions for aphasia improve language functions more than those by spontaneous recovery. Another significant effect is that these interventions help patients acquire communication techniques utilizing the remaining functions, thereby improving their quality of life.

Speech therapy approaches for aphasia are as follows: the therapeutic approach for functional deficits, the compensatory approach for disabilities, and the environment improvement approach for social disadvantages.

Examples of therapeutic approaches include Shuell's stimulus-facilitation approach [54], deblocking method [55], functional reorganization method [56], cognitive neuropsychological approach [57], semantic therapy [58], and melodic intonation therapy (MIT) [59]. They are considered effective for improving aphasia itself.

Meanwhile, examples of compensatory approaches for disabilities include acquisition practices for compensatory means, such as gesture practice, drawing practice, and practice for using other strategies, as well as practices for using compensatory means, such as the use of promoting aphasics' communicative effectiveness (PACE) and augmentative and alternative communication (AAC). In group therapy, patients with aphasia practice communicating effectively with other patients using available language and nonlanguage means [60, 61]. For patients with aphasia having communication difficulty at the onset, speech and language therapists must establish means of communication at early stages [62, 63].

Moreover, in addition to communication difficulty, patients with aphasia have various secondary problems in their daily lives, including difficulties in social connection, such as using financial institutions, public offices, public transportation systems, and commuting to the hospital. They also face problems, such as restrictions, in going to places for communicating with others and participating in leisure activities [64]. Simmons-Mackie et al. argued that encouraging the acquisition of communication partners promotes social participation among patients with aphasia and improves their communication skills. To resolve social and psychological issues among patients with aphasia, it is essential to promote family counseling and interactions with communication partners [65].

For rehabilitating patients with aphasia, it is desirable to appropriately approach the factors hindering communication and provide rehabilitation with a focus on life in the future.

Conflict of interest

The authors declare no conflict of interest.

Author details

Chiaki Yamaji* and Shinichiro Maeshima
Graduate School of Rehabilitation, Kinjo University, Hakusan, Japan

*Address all correspondence to: yamaji-c@fujita-hu.ac.jp

References

[1] Culton GL. Spontaneous recovery from Aphasia. Journal of Speech and Hearing Research. 1969;**12**(4).825-832

[2] Hartman J. Measurement of early spontaneous recovery from aphasia with stroke. Annals of Neurology. 1981;**9**(1): 89-91

[3] Lomas J, Kertesz A. Patterns of spontaneous recovery in aphasic groups: A study of adult stroke patients. Brain and Language. 1978;**5**(3):388-401

[4] Meshima S, Tanemura J, Shigeno K, Hasegawa T, Baba M, Imazu Y, et al. Natural recovery of aphasia due to cerebrovascular disorder. The Japanese Journal of Rehabilitation Medicine. 1992;**29**(2):123-130

[5] Lendrem W, Lincoln NB. Spontaneous recovery of language in patients with aphasia between 4 and 34 weeks after stroke. Journal of Neurology, Neurosurgery, and Psychiatry. 1985;**48**(8):743-748

[6] Sarno MT, Levita E. Natural course of recovery in severe aphasia. Archives of Physical Medicine and Rehabilitation. 1971;**52**(4):175-178

[7] Saur D, Lange R, Baumgaertner A, Schraknepper V, Willmes K, Rijntjes M, et al. Dynamics of language reorganization after stroke. Brain. 2006;**129**(6):1371-1384

[8] Heiss WD, Kessler J, Thiel A, Ghaemi M, Karbe H. Differential capacity of left and right hemispheric areas for compensation of poststroke aphasia. Annals of Neurology. 1999; **45**(4):430-438

[9] Mimura M, Kato M, Kato M, Sano Y, Kojima T, Naeser M, et al. Prospective and retrospective studies of recovery in aphasia. Changes in cerebral blood flow and language functions. Brain. 1998; **121**(11):2083-2094

[10] Pani E, Zheng X, Wang J, Norton A, Schlaug G. Right hemisphere structures predict poststroke speech fluency. Neurology. 2016;**86**(17):1574-1581

[11] Laska AC, Hellblom A, Murray V, Kahan T, Von Arbin M. Aphasia in acute stroke and relation to outcome. Journal of Internal Medicine. 2001;**249**(5): 413-422

[12] Sands E, Sarno MT, Shankweiler D. Long-term assessment of language function in aphasia due to stroke. Archives of Physical Medicine and Rehabilitation. 1969;**50**(4):202-206

[13] Vignolo LA. Evolution of aphasia and language rehabilitation: A retrospective exploratory study. Cortex: A Journal Devoted to the Study of the Nervous System and Behavior. 1964; **1**(3):344-367

[14] REhabilitation and recovery of peopLE with Aphasia after StrokE (RELEASE) Collaborators. Predictors of poststroke Aphasia recovery: A systematic review-informed individual participant data meta-analysis. Stroke. 2021;**52**(5):1778-1787

[15] Meinzer M, Harnish S, Conway T, Crosson B. Recent developments in functional and structural imaging of aphasia recovery after stroke. Aphasiology. 2011;**25**(3):271-290

[16] Pedersen PM, Jørgensen HS, Nakayama H, Raaschou HO, Olsen TS. Aphasia in acute stroke: Incidence, determinants, and recovery. Annals of Neurology. 1995;**38**(4):659-666

[17] Pedersen PM, Vinter K, Olsen TS. Aphasia after stroke: Type, severity and prognosis. CED. 2004;**17**(1):35-43

[18] Lazar RM, Speizer AE, Festa JR, Krakauer JW, Marshall RS. Variability in language recovery after first-time

stroke. Journal of Neurology, Neurosurgery, and Psychiatry. 2008; **79**(5):530-534

[19] Kertesz A. What do we learn from recovery from aphasia? Advances in Neurology. 1988;**47**:277-292

[20] Watila MM, Balarabe SA. Factors predicting post-stroke aphasia recovery. Journal of the Neurological Sciences. 2015;**352**(1-2):12-18

[21] Plowman E, Hentz B, Ellis C. Post-stroke aphasia prognosis: A review of patient-related and stroke-related factors. Journal of Evaluation in Clinical Practice. 2012;**18**(3):689-694

[22] Porch BE, Collins M, Wertz RT, Friden TP. Statistical prediction of change in aphasia. Journal of Speech and Hearing Research. 1980;**23**(2): 312-321

[23] Pickersgill MJ, Lincoln NB. Prognostic indicators and the pattern of recovery of communication in aphasic stroke patients. Journal of Neurology, Neurosurgery, and Psychiatry. 1983; **46**(2):130-139

[24] Basso A, Capitani E, Vignolo LA. Influence of rehabilitation on language skills in Aphasic patients: A controlled study. Archives of Neurology. 1979; **36**(4):190-196

[25] Basso A, Capitani E, Moraschini S. Sex differences in recovery from aphasia. Cortex. 1982;**18**(3):469-475

[26] Pizzamiglio L, Mammucari A, Razzano C. Evidence for sex differences in brain organization in recovery in aphasia. Brain and Language. 1985; **25**(2):213-223

[27] Kansaku K, Kitazawa S. Imaging studies on sex differences in the lateralization of language. Neuroscience Research. 2001;**41**(4):333-337

[28] Shaywitz BA, Shaywitz SE, Pugh KR, Constable RT, Skudlarski P, Fulbright RK, et al. Sex differences in the functional organization of the brain for language. Nature. 1995;**373**(6515): 607-609

[29] Kertesz A, McCabe P. Recovery patterns and prognosis in aphasia. Brain. 1977;**100**(Pt 1):1-18

[30] Butfield E, Zangwill OL. Re-education in aphasia; a review of 70 cases. Journal of Neurology, Neurosurgery, and Psychiatry. 1946;**9**(2):75-79

[31] Knecht S, Dräger B, Deppe M, Bobe L, Lohmann H, Flöel A, et al. Handedness and hemispheric language dominance in healthy humans. Brain. 2000;**123**(12):2512-2518

[32] Benson DF. Aphasia, Alexia and Agraphia. New York: Churchill Livingstone; 1980. p. 226

[33] Albert ML, Goodglass H, Helm NA, Rubens AB, Alexander MP. Heidelberg: Clinical Aspects of Dysphasia. Heidelberg: Springer Science & Business Media; 2013. p. 201

[34] Subirana A. The prognosis in aphasia in relation to cerebral dominance and handedness. Brain. 1958;**81**(3):415-425

[35] Brown JR, Simonson J. A clinical study of 100 aphasic patients. 1. Observations on lateralization and localization of lesions. Neurology. 1957;7(11):777-783

[36] Smith A. Objective indices of severity of chronic aphasia in stroke patients. The Journal of Speech and Hearing Disorders. 1971;**36**(2):167-207

[37] Assal G, Perentes E, Deruaz JP. Crossed aphasia in a right-handed patient. Postmortem findings. Archives of Neurology. 1981 Jul;**38**(7):455-458

[38] Hammond GR, Kaplan RJ. Language lateralization and handedness: Estimates based on clinical data. Brain and Language. 1982;**16**(2):348-351

[39] Anastasopoulos G, Kokkini D. Cerebral dominance and localisation of the language functions. ENE. 1962; **143**(1):6-19

[40] Davis GA. Incorporating parameters of natural conversation in aphasia treatment. In: Language Intervention Strategies in Adult Aphasia. Baltimore: Williams and Wilkins; 1981. pp. 169-193

[41] Demeurisse G, Demol O, Derouck M, de Beuckelaer R, Coekaerts MJ, Capon A. Quantitative study of the rate of recovery from aphasia due to ischemic stroke. Stroke. 1980;**11**(5):455-458

[42] Hartman J. Measurement of early spontaneous recovery from aphasia with stroke. Annals of Neurology. 1981;**9**(1): 89-91

[43] Mohr JP, Sidman M, Stoddard LT, Leicester J, Rosenberger PB. Evolution of the deficit in total aphasia. Neurology. 1973;**23**(12):1302-1312

[44] Bakheit AMO, Shaw S, Carrington S, Griffiths S. The rate and extent of improvement with therapy from the different types of aphasia in the first year after stroke. Clinical Rehabilitation. 2007;**21**:941-949

[45] Maeshima S, Okamoto S, Okazaki H, Funahashi R, Hiraoka S, Hori H, et al. Aphasia following left putaminal hemorrhage at a rehabilitation hospital. European Neurology. 2018;**79**(1-2):33-37

[46] Marchina S, Zhu LL, Norton A, Zipse L, Wan CY, Schlaug G. Impairment of speech production predicted by lesion load of the left arcuate fasciculus. Stroke. 2011;**42**(8): 2251-2256

[47] Lincoln NB, McGuirk E, Mulley GP, Lendrem W, Jones AC, Mitchell JR. Effectiveness of speech therapy for aphasic stroke patients. A randomised controlled trial. Lancet. 1984;**1**(8388): 1197-1200

[48] Levita E. Effects of speech therapy on aphasics' responses to functional communication profile. Perceptual and Motor Skills. 1978;**47**(1):151-154

[49] Wertz RT, Weiss DG, Aten JL, Brookshire RH, García-Buñuel L, Holland AL, et al. Comparison of clinic, home, and deferred language treatment for aphasia. A veterans administration cooperative study. Archives of Neurology. 1986;**43**(7):653-658

[50] Maeshima S, Okamoto S, Sonoda S, Osawa A. Data analysis of recovery from aphasia with stroke. Higher Brain Function Research. 2014;**34**(3): 298-304

[51] Cicerone KD, Dahlberg C, Malec JF, Langenbahn DM, Felicetti T, Kneipp S, et al. Evidence-based cognitive rehabilitation: Updated review of the literature from 1998 through 2002. Archives of Physical Medicine and Rehabilitation. 2005;**86**(8):1681-1692

[52] Mimura M, Sano Y, Tateishi M, Tanemura J. A Meta-Analysis of clinical outcomes in the treatment aphasia in Japan. Higher Brain Function Research. 2010;**30**(1):42-52

[53] Brady MC, Kelly H, Godwin J, Enderby P, Campbell P. Speech and language therapy for aphasia following stroke. Cochrane Database of Systematic Reviews. 2016;(6) No.CD000425. DOI: 10.1002/14651858.CD000425.pub4

[54] Shuell H, Jenkins JJ, Jimenez-Pabbn E. Aphasia in Adults. New York: Hoeber Medical/ Harper & Row; 1964

[55] Weigl E. The phenomenon of temporary deblocking in Aphasia. STUF -

Language Typology and Universals. 1961;**14**(1-4):337-364

[56] Luria AR. Osnoby neiropskihologii. Moskva: MGU; 1973

[57] Pinto-Grau M, O'Connor S, Murphy L, Costello E, Heverin M, Vajda A, et al. Validation and standardization of the Psycholinguistic Assessments of Language Processing in Aphasia (PALPA). Aphasiology. DOI: 10.1080/02687038.2020.1836317

[58] Howard D, Patterson K, Franklin S, Orchard-Lisle V, Morton J. Treatment of word retrieval deficits in aphasia. A comparison of two therapy methods. Brain. 1985;**108**(4):817-829

[59] Albert ML, Sparks RW, Helm NA. Melodic intonation therapy for aphasia. Archives of Neurology. 1973;**29**(2):130-131

[60] Elman RJ, Bernstein-Ellis E. The efficacy of group communication treatment in adults with chronic aphasia. Journal of Speech, Language, and Hearing Research. 1999;**42**(2): 411-419

[61] Dahlberg CA, Cusick CP, Hawley LA, Newman JK, Morey CE, Harrison-Felix CL, et al. Treatment efficacy of social communication skills training after traumatic brain injury: A randomized treatment and deferred treatment controlled trial. Archives of Physical Medicine and Rehabilitation. 2007;**88**(12):1561-1573

[62] Herrmann M, Reichle T, Lucius-Hoene G, Wallesch CW, Johannsen-Horbach H. Nonverbal communication as a compensative strategy for severely nonfluent aphasics? A quantitative approach. Brain and Language. 1988;**33**(1):41-54

[63] Helm-Estabrooks N, Fitzpatrick PM, Barresi B. Visual action therapy for global aphasia. The Journal of Speech and Hearing Disorders. 1982;**47**(4):385-389

[64] Dorze GL, Brassard C. A description of the consequences of aphasia on aphasic persons and their relatives and friends, based on the WHO model of chronic diseases. Aphasiology. 1995;**9**(3):239-255

[65] Simmons-Mackie N, Raymer A, Cherney LR. Communication partner training in Aphasia: An updated systematic review. Archives of Physical Medicine and Rehabilitation. 2016;**97**(12):2202-2221

Chapter 6

Treatment Approaches for Word Retrieval Deficits in Persons with Aphasia: Recent Advances

Deepak Puttanna, Akshaya Swamy, Sathyapal Puri Goswami and Abhishek Budiguppe Panchakshari

Abstract

Word retrieval deficit is found to be one of the most persistent symptoms reported among the constellation of symptoms exhibited by persons with aphasia (PWAs). This deficit restraints the persons with aphasia to perform with ease across day-to-day conversations. As a consequence, PWAs fail to communicate their desired ideas or thoughts. Word retrieval is an intricate process as it entails various levels of processing. In addition, word retrieval breakdown can occur at multiple levels (semantic level or lexical-semantic level, or phonological level). Thus, there is a need for speech-language pathologists (SLPs) to treat this deficit through effective treatment approaches. In recent decades, semantic feature analysis, verb network strengthening treatment, and phonological component analysis have received greater focus and importance in treating word retrieval deficits. Many studies confirmed that the use of these treatment approaches on PWAs possesses a pivotal role in remediating word retrieval deficits.

Keywords: word retrieval, lexical-semantic strengthening, semantic therapy, phonological therapy

1. Introduction

Word retrieval deficits remain one of the enduring symptoms in most PWAs [1]. Word retrieval deficits are events where the individual exhibits word-finding difficulty in conversation or while conveying their ideas or thoughts. The prevailing literature on word retrieval failures suggests that this deficit varies in their cognitive and neural underpinnings among discrete variants of aphasia. The SLP treating word retrieval deficits firstly needs to understand the nature of word retrieval breakdown (semantic or phonemic). These are ascertained *via* comprehensive naming assessments, and then based on the nature of word retrieval failures, appropriate treatment paradigms need to be employed.

2. Pathophysiology of naming impairments

The word retrieval process is an intricate process requiring two critical stages—semantic and phonologic [2, 3]. The retrieval process is strongly influenced by the modality in which they receive the input. For instance, confrontation picture naming involves object recognition as the primary input mechanism, followed by activation of the semantic system. The semantic system aids in storing the meaning and has associated information about the activated word. Finally, the semantic system activates modality-specific output lexicons for spoken, written words, and actions. With respect to spoken naming, lexical phonological output systems are activated. Subsequent to semantic and phonologic lexical retrieval stages, the post-lexical and articulatory process aids in the planning and execution of the verbal responses. These complex processes involved in word retrieval are likely to be affected in individuals with brain insult resulting in word retrieval impairment.

The word retrieval breakdown associated with PWAs is mediated by a distributed left hemisphere neural network (Hart & Kraut, 2007). There is a large body of evidence that suggests a lesion in the inferior temporal cortex is responsible for word retrieval impairments. Indeed, these impairments may vary with respect to the grammatical class and the impairments may be more for nouns than for verbs [4–6]. The lexical phonological output is mediated *via* the left superior temporal gyrus and inferior parietal cortex [1]. Lesions noted at the left frontal operculum result in non-fluent forms of aphasia, which result in difficulty in retrieving verbs than nouns [4–6]. Wilshire and Coslett [7] opine that word retrieval impairment can be accredited as an interface between syntactic and lexical processes. As far as the brain structure affected is concerned, the thalamus plays an indispensable role in word retrieval; as a result, lesions at the thalamus result in word retrieval impairment also [8].

3. Treatment approaches

Most of the treatment protocols developed for discrete variants of aphasia address the domains of linguistic deficit in aphasia. This implies that the protocol would be merely beneficial for semantically related deficits or phonological-based deficits. Traditionally, treatment rendered to PWAs relies on a symptomatic approach. Owing to the fact, aphasia is a multifaceted condition and entails the complex nature of the processing, and treatment for PWAs is explained along a continuum of naturalness [9].

One end of the continuum is the participation-based or socially oriented approach that primarily focuses on naturalness. Under this domain, the life participation approach [10] is streamlined as a socially oriented approach. LPAA aids in re-engagement of life to maximize an individual's quality of life and communication skills. The other hand of the continuum is the impaired-based approach. The impaired-based approach works on the premise of enhancing individuals' linguistic abilities. Subsequently, the treatment paradigms related to it were designed with the rationale of obviating the damaged processes.

3.1 Impaired-based approach

Impaired-based word retrieval paradigms are deployed to maximize the word retrieval abilities in contexts of speech and conversation. In the recent past, various types of word retrieval paradigms have been meticulously developed to remediate retrieval deficits. These are some of the seminal word retrieval paradigms, for instance, cueing hierarchy, phonological component analysis (PCA), semantic feature analysis (SFA), and Verb Network Strengthening Treatment (VNeST).

3.2 Cueing hierarchies

In cueing hierarchy paradigm, the SLP renders a series of discrete and potent cues to facilitate the targeted word. When PWAs retrieve the desired target word, the clinician encourages to repeat the target word several times, or the clinician presents cues in reverse order until the PWA provides the desired response. While using cueing hierarchy in PWAs, SLPs must ensure the more and less effective cues pertaining to the individual. In this paradigm, the targeted word is elicited through both semantic and phonological cues.

However, few studies highlight the potent role of semantics over phonological cues or vice versa (e.g., [11–13]). A review study by Patterson (2001) was carried out to uncover the effectiveness of cueing hierarchy in remediating word retrieval failures. The consolidated reports by various studies posit that cueing hierarchy paradigm aids in showing ameliorated performance for the trained words with various levels of retrieval deficits (semantic or phonological).

There are few interesting studies, which appraised the effectiveness of cueing hierarchy paradigm by inculcating variations in the training. Marshall, Karow, Freed, and Babcock [14] compared the effect of personalized cues (i.e., a phrase developed by the individuals themselves) over phonological cues. The findings computed in the study showed that individuals using personalized semantic information (e.g., "Apple is red in color"? or the animal which eats flesh?) outperformed phonological cues alone. Furthermore, the cueing paradigm was trained and developed through software to provide more flexibility and to reach a large population who are deprived of receiving speech-language therapy services.

Over the recent decades, researchers have used a computerized version of cueing hierarchy paradigm. The finding of the study evinced ameliorated performance for the trained words in moderate–severe naming impaired individuals [15, 16].

3.3 Phonological component analysis (PCA)

PCA is one of the renowned treatment approaches to remediate word retrieval deficits [17]. This approach emphasizes the use of self-cueing. In PCA therapy, individuals are presented with a picture placing at the center of the chart, and then, they are asked to name the corresponding picture. Simultaneously, PWAs are asked to identify the phonological components such as rhyming words, the first sound, first sound associate, final sound, and the number of syllables with respect to the target word (**Figure 1**). While identifying the phonological cues, if individuals fail to produce desired responses, then they are given an array of choices (up to three choices). Out of these choices, individuals need to select one of the choices among three. Choices are presented *via* letter cards, and the clinician reads these choices aloud. The response elicited is noted in the chart. Once the response generation for each phonological component is complete, PWAs are able to retrieve the target item independently. When they generate the desired response, then positive feedback is provided. Considering the possibilities of errors, the clinician models the desired response and needs reiteration by PWAs.

The impact of PCA treatment on word retrieval skills per se has been studied in many research studies. The evidences from these studies seem to be conducive as they manifest ameliorated performance in trained items in most of the studies [18, 19]. On the other hand, the findings for PCA on untrained stimuli seem to be less robust. Thus, researchers posit poor generalization skills following PCA treatment [11, 18].

3.4 Semantic feature analysis (SFA)

3.4.1 SFA for objects

SFA intends to manifest ameliorated performance in lexical retrieval abilities per se in PWAs. This treatment systematically trains the target word by activating the

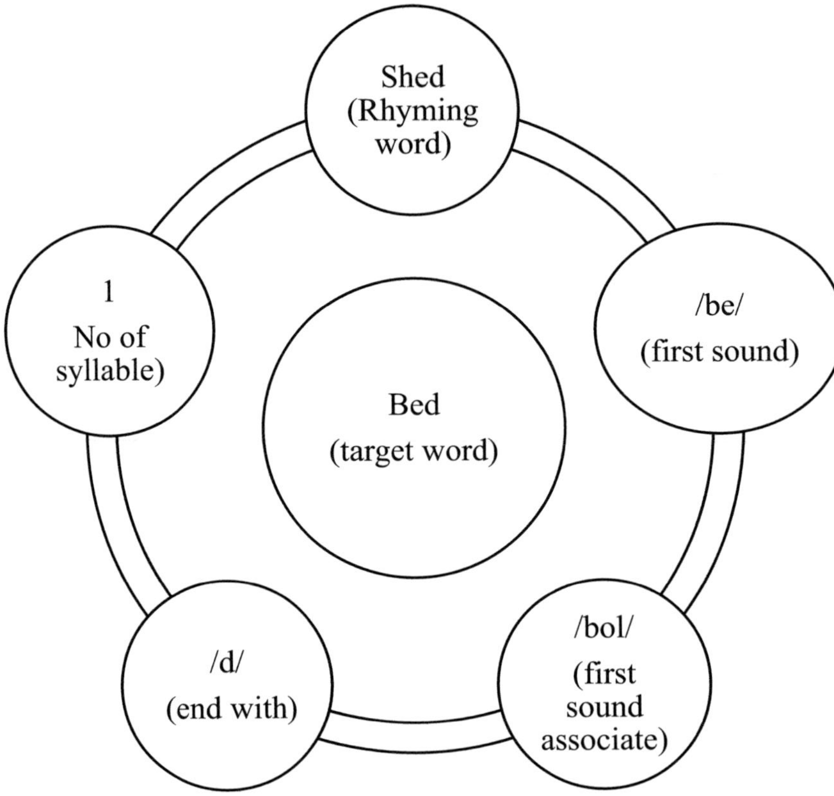

Figure 1.
Flowchart depicting the procedure of phonological component analysis (PCA) treatment.

discrete semantic attributes, enhancing the semantic networks corresponding to the target word. In this treatment, the clinician places a target word picture card in the center of the chart. The chart comprises the discrete semantic features—superordinate category, use, action, physical properties, location, and association of the corresponding target word (**Figure 2**). In short, the clinician initially provides the target picture; subsequently, PWAs will be asked to retrieve the corresponding semantic attributes. If PWAs fail to name, then the clinician cues them to retrieve the desired responses. To provide semantic features, the clinician reads the printed cues and provides the relevant features both orally and in written forms. The semantic feature generation aids in distinguishing desired features versus undesired features of the target word. Initially, SFA training emphasizes maximal cueing by the clinician. Eventually, cueing is faded as the training progresses. The semantic features enhance the activation of the corresponding target word; consequently, PWAs name the items without any cues. If PWAs are not able to retrieve the target item and corresponding features, then the clinician delivers the name and features [20].

3.4.2 SFA for verbs

Semantic feature analysis treatment for verbs follows a slightly distinct protocol compared to noun training. In this treatment, a picture of the target action will be placed at the center of the chart. The PWA will be asked to retrieve the corresponding action. If they fail, the clinician cues the action verb using the following semantic features—(a) the agent/experiencer of the action ("Who usually does

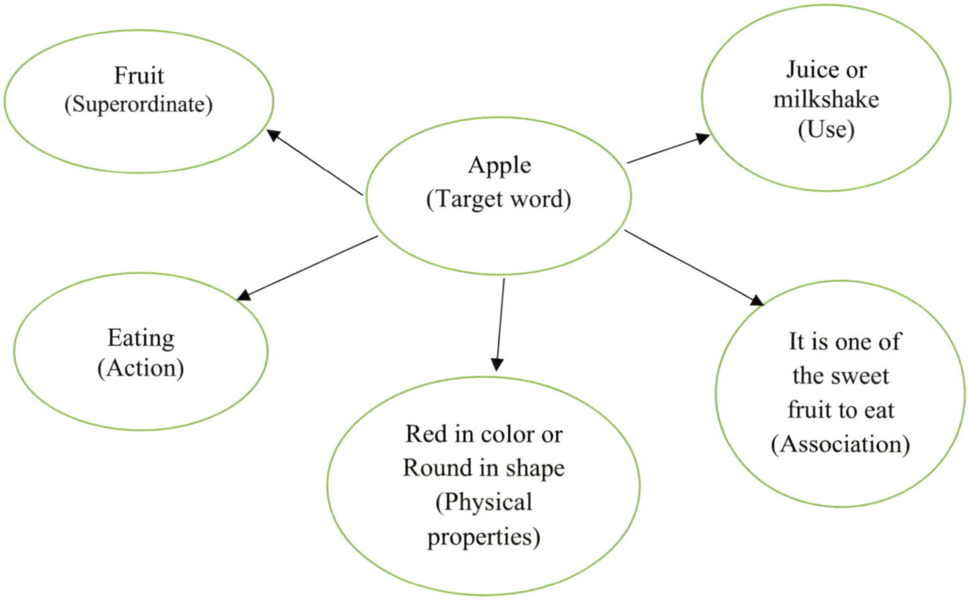

Figure 2.
Flowchart depicting SFA treatment for noun.

this?"), the theme/patient ("On what/ by whom is it performed?"), the location ("Where does this action happen?"), the purpose of the action ("Why does this happen?"), the means of carrying out the action ("What part of the body or what tool is used to make this happen?"), and the related objects or actions that reminded the participant of the target verb ("What does it make you think of?"). These features were introduced one at a time and in the same order mentioned above. The PWA's response will be noted down. If the PWA failed to provide the desired response, then the clinician prompts a response. The prompts can be either semantic or phonological. After generating all six semantic features, the PWAs are asked to name the target action without any prompts. Despite these prompts, if the PWA still fails to arrive at desired responses, then the clinician delivers the target action word. The PWA is asked to repeat the action word after the clinician models. Finally, they will be asked to construct a simple sentence using the verb; if they are unable to produce, then the clinician assists in constructing simple sentences or narrating the simple sentences for PWAs. The PWA is prompted to repeat after the clinician narrates the sentence (**Figure 3**).

Further, to document SFA treatment findings across various studies, a systematic review was conducted [21]. This review study pooled data from 21 studies consisting of 55 PWAs encompassed both fluent and nonfluent variants of aphasia. The findings revealed robust findings for 45 out of 55 PWAs for the trained items; 32 out of 55 PWAs were able to maintain the responses. In addition, 40% of PWAs were able to manifest generalization of response to the untrained stimuli. The SFA treatment manifested robust outcomes for fluent and mild–moderate severity of aphasia compared to nonfluent and severe forms of aphasia [22–25]. Overall, SFA is deemed as a viable treatment approach in the diminution of word retrieval deficits. In light of these findings, future studies on SFA should focus on observing or noting the generalization on untrained stimuli. A future implication would be that the treatment approach can be extended by documenting the improvement in the discourse genre.

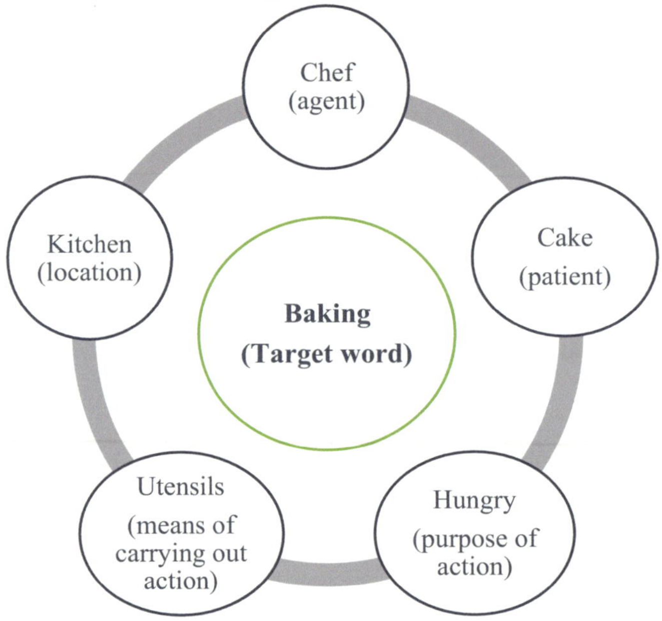
Chef
(agent)
Cake
(patient)
Hungry
(purpose of action)
Utensils
(means of carrying out action)
Kitchen
(location)
Baking
(Target word)

Figure 3.
Flowchart depicting SFA treatment for verbs.

3.5 Verb network strengthening treatment (VNeST)

VNeST was developed on the premise that if treatment paradigms utilized verbs as the core element then it can aid in the activation of a wide array of semantic networks. In addition, it may assist in the construction of simple active sentences. VNeST protocol constitutes a total of six steps to remediate word retrieval deficits [26]. These steps are as follows:

1. *Step one—Generation of Verb, Agent, and Patient*: In this step, the clinician probes PWAs to retrieve the verb with the relevant semantic cues. If they are unable to retrieve the target verb, then maximal cueing is provided. Subsequently, PWA will be probed to elicit relevant agents (doer of the action) and patients (receiver of the action) for the intended verb. If PWA fails to elicit the corresponding agent and patient pairs on their own, then they will be provided with a series of choices (maximum cues).

   To illustrate, to retrieve the verb "Baking," the following semantic cues can be used: (a) This is usually done in the kitchen; (b) this is usually done using utensils/stove; (c) this is usually done to prepare bread, cake. For identification of the corresponding agent for the verb "Bake," individuals will be provided with choices (written cards) of photographer, farmer, and chef. PWA will be asked to identify the corresponding agent for the verb "Bake." Eventually, a similar cueing strategy will be carried out for the identification of the patient. In addition, PWA will be encouraged to produce agents and patients from their experiences. The rationale of step one is that eliciting a wide array of agent/patient pairs may promote the activation of discrete semantic networks corresponding to the verb.

2. *Step two—Reading the Agent/ Patient Pairs*: In this step, the PWA is prompted to read the generated agent/patient pairs corresponding verb. If they fail to read the simple sentence, then the choral reading strategy is employed.

3. *Step three—Response to Wh Questions:* The clinician intends to expand the generated agent/patient pairs in this step. That is, PWA is probed with series of "Wh" questions related to the pairs. However, this expansion is confounded to only one pair of agents/patients.

4. *Step four —Judgment*: This step is focused on carrying out sentence judgment by the varying agent or patient order. Four combinations of sentences will be presented/read to the PWA—(a) inappropriate agent form (doctor baked cake), (b) inappropriate patient form (chef baked tree), (c) sentence reversal (cake baked chef), and (d) the appropriate form (chef baked cake). The PWA has to judge where each sentence is correct or incorrect. Both steps *three* and *four* focus on strengthening the relationship among the verbs and their corresponding agent/patient pairs.

5. *Step five—Independent Retrieval of Verb:* In this step, the PWA has to retrieve the verb without any cues. If they are unable to retrieve, then prompts are provided.

6. *Step six—Independent Retrieval of Agent/Patient:* This step intends to elicit agent/patient pair for the target verb independently. Here, no prompts or cues will be rendered. This step aids in strengthening the discussed pairs before moving into the successive trained stimuli.

The relevance of steps with respect to the activation system occurring in the VNeST protocol is depicted in **Figure 4**.

In order to understand the effectiveness of VNeST treatment, Edmonds [27] conducted a review study. A total of 19 English-speaking PWAs received VNeST treatment across different studies [26, 28–30]. These studies enrolled PWAs who evinced chronic aphasia with severity ranging between mild and severe form; PWAs showed no impairment or moderate impairment in cognitive-linguistic quick test and had good comprehension scores. Ten verbs were trained. The PWAs enrolled in these studies were trained for 4–15 weeks, twice a week (each session would last for 3–3.5 hours), wherein the majority of PWAs received training for 10 weeks on an average. On the other hand, Furnas and Edmonds [29] provided training thrice a week, with each session would last for 2 hours per session for the time interval

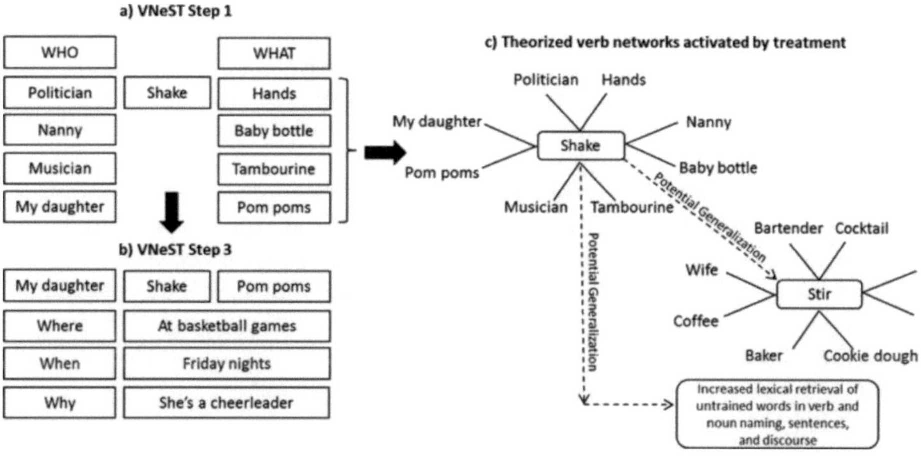

Figure 4.
Activation of the semantic network using VNeST treatment protocol. Edmonds [27].

of six weeks. Outcomes of this review study served as the preliminary evidence. These studies posit that VNeST training reinforces lexical retrieval at a single word, sentence, and discourse genre across discrete variants of aphasia and with different levels of severity.

In addition, these studies evinced improvement in functional communication, per se. The studies based on VNeST showed ameliorated performance in noun and verb naming, sentence production, and discourse genre across the trained and untrained conditions. Despite these prominent findings, more research is warranted to strengthen these findings. The majority of the studies showed mixed findings while gauging the generalization effect. Equivocal findings were also noted across fluent and nonfluent aphasia and across different levels of severity. These literatures failed to evince the specific pattern or mechanism responsible for showing improvement in specific types of aphasia. Thus, the VNeST training has to be assessed in detail for each type of aphasia.

4. Conclusions

This chapter focuses on some of the word retrieval treatment approaches. These approaches are mainly intended to ameliorate word representation and also to activate the phonological encoding stage of word retrieval. While gauging the effectiveness of any treatment approach, several factors are to be looked upon, namely—(1) maintenance of word retrieval skills per se followed by therapy; (2) response generalization to the untrained conditions and different treatment settings. The treatments discussed in this chapter discerned fairly good generalization and response maintenance in almost all the approaches. However, relatively poor generalization skills are noted in the PCA. Poor responses can be attributed to being surface-level training and redundancy of cues. In cases of more severe word retrieval deficits, the treatment paradigms discussed may not be suitable for the initial phase of treatment. Instead, the clinician must start the treatment with more direct facilitative treatment and gradually progress to the treatment that entails self-generation of words. Owing to this, speech-language pathologists should consider severity before selecting the specific word retrieval treatment.

Commonly raised concern in the treatment-related studies is the superiority of one treatment approach over the other or anyone specific treatment approach is engendered to show maximal benefits. The answers to these questions are still at preliminary levels, and these need to be documented by conducting various research on these lines. To our understanding, in the current scenario, no particular treatment approach is deemed as superior over other treatment approaches at a more advanced level. However, based on the prevailing evidence, the VNeST approach can be claimed as the streamlined approach compared to SFA and PCA at the surface level in remediating word retrieval deficits.

Word retrieval treatments needed to be selected meticulously, and their impact on functional communication needs to be looked into, as word retrieval deficits are engendered to evince a tremendous impact on the day-to-day conversation. In some word retrieval treatments, improvement may be confounded to trained conditions, or improvement may be generalized to few untrained conditions. Owing to this, treatment paradigms selected should include strategies that would aid the PWAs to show improvement even in the functional communication per se.

Author details

Deepak Puttanna[1]*, Akshaya Swamy[2], Sathyapal Puri Goswami[2] and Abhishek Budiguppe Panchakshari[3]

1 Father Muller College of Speech and Hearing, Mangalore, India

2 All India Institute of Speech and Hearing, Mysore, India

3 Nitte College of Speech and Hearing, Mangalore, India

*Address all correspondence to: deepakaryan064@gmail.com

References

[1] Goodglass H, Wingfield A. *Anomia: Neuroanatomical and Cognitive Correlates*. San Diego: Academic Press; 1997

[2] Hillis AE, Newhart M. Cognitive neuropsychological approaches to treatment of language disorder: introduction. In: Chapey R, editor. Language intervention strategies in aphasia and related neurogenic communication disorders. 5th ed. Baltimore: Lippincott Williams & Wilkins; 2008. pp. 595-606

[3] Nickels L. Spoken word production. In: *The Handbook of Cognitive Neuropsychology: What Deficits Reveal About the Human Mind*. Philadelphia: Psychology Press; 2001. pp. 291-320

[4] Damasio AR, Tranel D. Nouns and verbs are retrieved with differently distributed neural systems. Proceedings of the National Academy of Sciences. 1993;*90*(11):4957-4960

[5] Hillis AE, Tuffiash E, Wityk RJ, Barker PB. Regions of neural dysfunction associated with impaired naming of actions and objects in acute stroke. Cognitive Neuropyschology. 2002;7:191-243

[6] Tranel D, Damasio H, Damasio AR. A neural basis for the retrieval of conceptual knowledge. Neuropsychologia. 1997;*35*(10): 1319-1327

[7] Wilshire CE, Coslett HB. *Disorder of word retrieval in aphasia*: theories and potential applications. In: Nadeau SE, Rothi LJG, Crosson B, editors. Aphasia and Language: Theory to Practice. New York: Guilford Press; 2000. pp. 82-107

[8] Raymer AM, Moberg P, Crosson B, Nadeau S, Rothi LG. Lexical–semantic deficits in two patients with dominant thalamic infarction. Neuropsychologia. 1997;*35*(2):211-219

[9] Paul R, Cascella PW. Introduction to clinical methods in communication disorders. Baltimore, MD: Brookes Publishing; 2007

[10] LPAA Project Group, Chapey, R., Duchan, J., Elman, R., Garcia, L, Kagan, A., Lyon J., & Simmons-Mackie, N. (2008). Life participation approach to aphasia: A statement of values for the future. In R. Chapey (Ed.), Language intervention strategies in aphasiaand related neurogenic communication disorders (5th ed.). Baltimore, MD: Lippincott, Williams & Wilkins

[11] Raymer AM, Thompson CK, Jacobs B, & Le Grand, H. R. Phonological treatment of naming deficits in aphasia: Model-based generalizationanalysis. Aphasiology. 1993;7(1):27-53

[12] Wambaugh, J. L., Doyle, P. J., Linebaugh, C. W., Spencer, K. A., & Kalinyak-Fliszar, M. (1999, October). Effects of deficit-oriented treatments on lexical retrieval in a patient with semantic and phonological deficits. In *Brain and Language* (Vol. 69, No. 3, pp. 446-450). 525 B ST, STE 1900, San Diego, CA, USA: Academic Press Inc

[13] Wambaugh JL, Linebaugh CW, Doyle PJ, Martinez AL, Kalinyak-Fliszar M, Spencer KA. Effects of two cueing treatments on lexical retrieval in aphasic speakers with different levels of deficit. Aphasiology. 2001;*15*(10-11):933-950

[14] Marshall RC, Karow CM, Freed DB, Babcock P. Effects of personalised cue form on the learning of subordinate category names by aphasic and non-brain-damaged subjects. Aphasiology. 2002;*16*(7):763-771

[15] Fink RB, Brecher A, Schwartz MF, Robey RR. A computer-implemented protocol for treatment of naming

disorders: Evaluation of clinician-guided and partially self-guided instruction. Aphasiology. 2002;*16* (10-11):1061-1086

[16] Ramsberger, G., & Marie, B. (2007). Self-administered cued naming therapy: A single-participant investigation of a computer-based therapy program replicated in four cases. American Speech Language Pathology. 16:343-58

[17] Howard DAVID, Patterson K, Franklin S, Orchard-Lisle V, Morton J. Treatment of word retrieval deficits in aphasia. Brain. 1985;*108*(8):17-829

[18] Hickin J, Best W, Herbert R, Howard D, Osborne F. Phonological therapy for word-finding difficulties: A re-evaluation. Aphasiology. 2002;*16*(10-11):981-999

[19] Greenwood A, Grassly J, Hickin J, Best W. Phonological and orthographic cueing therapy: A case of generalised improvement. Aphasiology. 2010;*24*(9):991-1016

[20] Boyle M. Semantic feature analysis treatment for aphasic word retrieval impairments: What's in a name? Topics in Stroke Rehabilitation. 2010;**17**(6): 411-422

[21] Efstratiadou EA, Papathanasiou I, Holland R, Archonti A, Hilari K. A systematic review of semantic feature analysis therapy studies for aphasia. Journal of Speech, Language, and Hearing Research. 2018;*61*(5): 1261-1278

[22] Antonucci SM. The use of semantic feature analysis in group aphasia treatment. Aphasiology. 2009;**23**: 854-866

[23] Boyle M. Semantic feature analysis treatment for anomia in two fluent aphasia syndromes. American Journal of Speech Language Pathology. 2004;**13**: 236-249

[24] Coelho CA, McHugh RE, Boyle, M. Semantic feature analysis as a treatment for aphasic dysnomia: A replication. Aphasiology. 2000;**14**(2):133-142

[25] Hashimoto N. The use of semantic- and phonological-based feature approaches to treat naming deficits in aphasia. Clinical Linguistics & Phonetics. 2012;**26**(6):518-553

[26] Edmonds LA, Nadeau SE, Kiran S. Effect of verb network strengthening treatment (VNeST) on lexical retrieval of content words in sentences in persons with aphasia. Aphasiology. 2009;**23**(3): 402-424

[27] Edmonds LA. A review of verb network strengthening treatment. Topics in Language Disorders. 2016; **36**(2):123-135

[28] Edmonds LA, Babb M. Effect of verb network strengthening treatment in moderate-to-severe aphasia. American Journal of Speech-Language Pathology. 2011;**20**:131-145

[29] Edmonds LA, Mammino K, Ojeda, J. Effect of verb network strengthening treatment (VNeST) in persons with aphasia: Extension and replication of previous findings. American Journal of Speech-Language Pathology. 2014;**23**(2):312-329

[30] Furnas DW, Edmonds, L. A. The effect of computerised Verb Network Strengthening Treatment on lexical retrieval in aphasia. Aphasiology. 2014;**28**(4):401-420

Chapter 7

The Importance of Aphasia Communication Groups

Marina Charalambous and Maria Kambanaros

Abstract

Chronic aphasia is linked to poor functional recovery, depression, and social isolation. In the exploration of the above factors, the role of aphasia communication groups has evolved. Aphasia communication groups for stroke survivors with chronic aphasia and their communication buddies are gaining clinical importance. Communication buddies can be family members, friends, carers, health professionals, and speech and language therapy students who serve as communication facilitators for each group member. Group members share experiences on stroke and aphasia by using technology/tablets and the total communication approach. The benefits or outcomes of group involvement are measured by assessment of functional communication, individual self-ratings of the impact of aphasia on communication, and quality of life after stroke. The use of the communication buddy system, total communication approach, and systematic evaluations enables therapists to measure the effectiveness and efficacy of communication groups in terms of functional communication, social inclusion, and quality of life.

Keywords: communication buddies, quality of life, aphasia communication groups

1. Introduction

Aphasia is an acquired communication impairment that impacts the ability to speak, understand, read, write, and carry out mathematical calculations [1]. It is caused by damage to the language networks in the brain usually after stroke but not only [2]. Aphasia is linked to poorer functional recovery [3], return to work [4], activities of daily living [5], depression [6], and social isolation [7].

Functional communication and social participation are impaired in aphasia, which brings about reduced confidence in communication [8]. This leads to reduced interactions with family and friends [9] and smaller social networks [10]. Although maintaining social interactions and friendship networks in the chronic phase of aphasia (greater than 6-months post brain injury) has been identified as an important goal in aphasia rehabilitation, this is not regularly addressed by aphasia clinicians [9].

Historical models of aphasia assessment and treatment have focused mainly on the person's linguistic competence [11]. Even though people with aphasia (PWA) may have successfully achieved their therapeutic goals in individual speech and language therapy sessions, they still struggle to use their new communication skills successfully in natural environments, e.g., with family members, close friends, and their therapist outside of the clinic/treatment environment [12]. Contemporary rehabilitation approaches pay increasing attention to the pragmatic competence and the overall functionality of communication of PWA via aphasia communication groups (ACGs) [13].

In the context of the International Classification of Functioning, Disability and Health (ICF) [14], biopsychosocial models of disability, and particularly the Life Participation Approach to Aphasia Project Group [15], interest in ACGs is increasing in both research and clinical settings [16]. ACGs provide psychosocial benefits to PWA, including increasing social participation and peer support [17].

1.1 Defining aphasia communication groups

Aphasia communication groups (ACGs) are defined as small groups of people with aphasia and their communication partners who interact with each other on a regular basis. These groups include PWA who can communicate in any accessible way, are aware of each other's presence and perceive themselves, and are perceived by others, as being members of a group [18]. *ACGs* are described as informal groups meaning that they are more erratic and spontaneous, and less constrained by formal structures and power relationships compared to formal groups (committees, boards etc.) [19].

While ACGs can focus on the impairment-based characteristics of aphasia, the nature of the group setting tends to elicit functional, naturalistic forms of communication [20]. The actions and subject matter of each communication group vary enormously and depend mainly on the goals and aspirations of the group members. Group members develop close relationships with each other in a natural and supporting environment, which promotes meaningful conversations with people who empathize with their difficulties. *ACGs* work on the "barriers" that make communication challenging for the person with aphasia and their communication partners, and on what communication tools members could use to improve communication [21]. The different methodological approaches used in ACGs such as learning events, personal stories, and patient narratives foster functional communication, active engagement, and mutual support [22–24].

The primary *aim* of the *ACGs* is to provide support for PWA on learning about aphasia, communication opportunities to promote living well with aphasia, and improve quality of life [20]. Another common *goal* is the understanding that aphasia can be a life-long condition, and that aphasia is a "family issue," impacting not only the person with aphasia [21]. The main *pillar* of ACGs is to create a supportive and safe environment for meaningful communication and social endeavors that encompass interactive functional communication activities [21]. *ACGs* promote full participation and engagement in activities of interest and are inclusive to all PWA irrespective of degree and severity of aphasia [25]. In fact, ACGs have been likened to a "*rope team*" [26]. The term "rope team" comes from the sport of mountain climbing. The rope team will tether themselves together for safety to help prevent falls. By establishing a rope team, individuals with aphasia are provided with a positive atmosphere for participation and communication without fear of judgment. In aphasia rehabilitation, a rope team can consist of other healthcare professionals and caregivers, but, more importantly, others with aphasia.

1.2 Communication quality in aphasia communication groups

ACGs should seek to make improvements in the communication quality of PWA. Based on the *Communication Quality Guidelines* of the Royal College of Speech and Language Therapists (RCSLT) [27], this is fostered when groups are EASIER:

1. ***Effective***: by delivering group activities that adhere to evidence-based practice and result in improved activity and participation outcomes for PWA, based on individual needs;

2. ***Accessible***: by delivering ACGs that is timely, geographically reasonable, and provided in a setting where skills and resources are appropriate to medical/rehabilitation needs;

3. ***Safe***: by delivering ACGs that minimize risks and harm to service users;

4. ***Individualized/client-centered***: by delivering ACGs that consider the preferences and aspirations of individual service users and their communities;

5. ***Equitable***: by delivering ACGs that do not vary in quality because of personal characteristics such as gender, race, ethnicity, geographical location, or socioeconomic status;

6. ***Resource-efficient***: by delivering ACGs in a manner that maximizes resource use.

1.3 Why are aphasia communication groups important to people with aphasia?

Loneliness and social inaccessibility in chronic aphasia lead to poor community and public engagement [9]. Aphasia communication groups are an opportunity for social participation [28] that promote community integration, broaden friendship circles, and improve social connectedness [29]. Without prospects for *good communication,* PWA struggle to learn about their condition, to achieve personal goals, make friends, and interact meaningfully – all fundamental for citizenship and humanity and central to improving quality of life [27]. All these principles are offered to PWA in a communication group setting as they are given opportunities to exercise their human right on how to be involved with decisions about their care, make choices about their daily life, create opportunities to communicate their needs and thoughts, understand and express their necessities in relation to their health and wellbeing whilst being treated with respect and dignity [27].

ACGs are important to PWA as they have a common *purpose*: to become familiar with aphasia symptoms, to share personal experiences, support and encourage each other, and get trained on how to establish successful functional communication [25]. In a review by Attard and colleagues [30] on consumer perspectives on community ACGs, the findings revealed that group attendance formed positive relations for PWA with others, gave purpose in life, promoted environmental mastery, autonomy, personal growth, and self-acceptance. According to Lanyon and colleagues [31], PWA perceive community aphasia-group participation to be beneficial to their ability to live well with aphasia. Peer-to-peer communication strategies, shared roles and responsibilities, and consultation regarding group objectives and processes provide group members with the opportunity to become active contributors, demonstrate competence, and have positive influence over the group [31]. During the qualitative investigation of the factors impacting participation and integration of PWA in aphasia community groups, Lanyon and colleagues [31] revealed seven important features:

1. *Balanced interactional patterns*: reflects the balance and equal share in interactions between group members and leaders. It is associated with equal turn-taking opportunities and the promotion of the appropriate sensitivity of the group leader toward group members.

2. *An open and non-hierarchical group environment*: relates to the maintenance of an interactional space that provides active consultation between peers and opportunities for the members to share roles and assume responsibilities (such as activities planning, assisting in message transfer, and organizing coffee breaks).

3. *Communication awareness and education among members*: demonstrates the need for group members to learn communication support strategies and aphasia training to understand and interact respectfully with their fellow members.

4. *Meaningful activity*: shows the constant need of group members for authentic interactions related to day-to-day life situations and life-sharing experiences with socially-focused activities.

5. *Ritual and structure*: group rituals such as formal welcomes, opportunities for sharing information, and involvement in the preparation of a coffee break are considered the foundation for enabling members, regardless of their prior experience with group processes, to intergrade within the group and feel that they participate in a relaxed and nonthreatening environment.

6. *Composition and group size*: both size and composition are central to the involvement of PWA within the group and may function as a bridge or barrier to their positive participation experience. ACGs with a mixed composition of people with a range of communication abilities are considered more beneficial for PWA with more severe communication difficulties. Also, smaller group size (3–4 members) fosters the creation of individual *identity* of each group member and promotes family and friendship-like endeavors. On the contrary, large groups (15 members) are challenging for PWA to interact with.

7. *Group leadership*: Group organizers and leaders play a crucial role in shaping the pattern of interaction, encouraging an engaging space, and modeling effective interaction. ACGs should equalize the power and status between leaders and the members by elevating the position of member peers to group leaders.

Aphasia communication groups' positive participation promotes *patient involvement* (PI) and elevates discussions on how aphasia impacts activities of daily living, social integration, and participation [32]. Azios et al. [9] propose a *codesign* model of intervention and research on friendship maintenance within aphasia communication groups, as a means of addressing the issues of social isolation and other personal concerns of PWA. The *Quality of Communication Life Scale* [33] suggests that "the more positive the personal and environmental factors, the more successful the [person's] communication acts, the better the quality of communication life" (p. 2). Taking into consideration the perspectives, needs, and experiences of PWA, as service users in ACGs, it is critical to use PI approaches and activities that will accelerate translation to real-world activities and promote functional interventions and strategies for living successfully with aphasia (activity and participation level 0 [14]). Positive effects of ACGs where PWA are actively involved in decision making, build confidence in PWA to express their needs, whereas research evidence demonstrates positive health benefits of building interpersonal relationships and community while being part of an ACG [20].

2. Setting up an aphasia communication group

2.1 Establishing ground rules

Before establishing an ACG, members should discuss and agree on the group's ground rules using a SIMPLE approach. The ACG and each group member should be:

Supportive – Ask caring questions; listen attentively to responses/others.
Inspirational – Reassure others that life gets better and not to give-up.
Motivational – Encourage action and acknowledge improvement.
Practical – Offer options, helpful tips, and information and access to resources.
Life-affirming – Not deny or devalue/trivialize the feelings of others.
Educational – Talk about what's worked for them and others; offer guidance/counsel, but without giving prescriptive advice.

2.2 Inclusion criteria

The general inclusion criteria for *ACGs* are that PWA:

- are living in the community.
- have been discharged from acute and sub-acute rehabilitation.
- are in the chronic stage of aphasia.
- do not need additional medical support while being at the group.
- have given written informed consent to participate.
- have signed a confidentiality contract so they do not share the personal experiences and narratives of other group members with people outside the group.
- present with various types and severities of aphasia.

The inclusion criteria are usually adjusted according to the setting and the purpose of each ACG [21].

2.3 Group features

A successful group requires several features to be efficient: the members, the group, and the tasks/activities, the context [34]:

- The *Members*:
    - work cooperatively and not competitively.
    - support each other and show empathy.
    - get rewarded collectively and not individually.
    - are aware of the nature of the group process.

- The *Group*:
  - is relatively small (maximum five people).
  - is autonomous to address its activities and tasks.
  - has an effective leader/facilitator.
  - operates in the context of a supportive organization or community.
- The *Tasks/Activities*:
  - are accessible to all members.
  - are designed considering the individual skills of each member.
  - promote the active engagement of all members.
  - have precise objectives.
  - have a beginning and a defined end.
  - have measurable indicators of success.
- The *Context*:
  - The physical environment should be accessible.
  - Time schedule and agenda should be defined.
  - Resources should be allocated before enrolment.
  - External factors should be taken into consideration (traveling, financial issues).

2.4 Total communication

Group members practice total communication skills, i.e., gestures, singing, drawing, and writing, and/or a combination of all the above [20]. The main topics of discussion are learning about/refreshing knowledge on stroke and aphasia, linking the information to members' own experiences, asking questions, and discussing living with stroke and aphasia [21]. It is also important for members to share stories about life before the stroke [35]. Resources for total communication such as writing boards, notebooks, tables, communication books, aphasia friendly materials [36], and the Internet should be used to access information online [37].

2.5 Virtual aphasia communication groups

Group meetings can be established with face-to-face contact or digitally. Virtual group meetings and videoconferencing are a growing trend in aphasia rehabilitation with a major impact [38]. Online groups favor the person with mild to moderate aphasia, the member who is well motivated to participate and seeks interaction despite the means. In online ACGs, it is mandatory that members know how to operate a tablet, mobile phone, or a laptop independently and understand the ethics and procedures behind video conferencing [39]. Realistically, ACGs via video conferencing compared to face-to-face interaction need more time to plan and prepare. When technical problems occur, and they often do occur, they cause anxiety and frustration to the group. Some members become diverted into "fixing" the problem where others "switch off" from participating, factors that make the interaction dysfunctional. The experience of engaging in an online meeting is more mentally demanding as members must concentrate simultaneously on the content of the meeting, the visual material, and the constant input from several sources. Additionally, nonverbal cues are not detected easily, and the facilitator must be proactive in giving cues and prepare digital material to promote engagement.

3. Setting client-centered goals in the aphasia communication groups

According to Worrall and colleagues [40], goal setting in ACGs with PWA can be challenging because of members:

- *persisting language impairment* that makes expressing needs and discussion of experiences a long and demanding process.
- *cognitive difficulties* that create struggles with decision-making,
- strain in understanding the *abstract concept of aphasia.*
- *poor awareness* of their overall condition.
- feelings of *disempowerment* that arise when communication is distracted.
- *age as* members that are often older expect to be directed in one-on-one therapy rather than group treatment.

A further challenge is related to the *setting* that may reinforce a culture in which SLTs focus on the language impairment and are in control.

3.1 SMART short-term goals

At the beginning of each ACG, goals are discussed with the members of the group, which are more likely to be their long-term goals for aphasia rehabilitation in general. The facilitator along with the communication buddies needs to support the members of the group to break down these goals into SMART short-term goals that can be addressed in the group. These goals should be SMART: Specific, Measurable, Attainable, Relevant, and Time-based (**Figure 1**).

3.2 The SMARTER framework

In combination with the SMART goals, the SMARTER "Shared, Monitored, Accessible, Relevant, Transparent, Evolving, Relationship" framework encourages aphasia rehabilitation specialists engaged in group therapy to share the goal-setting process with the person with aphasia [41]. The procedure of setting SMARTER goals should be accomplished in a way that is accessible to the members of the group and ensures that the goals evolve with the needs of the clients. Within this framework, the person with aphasia is actively engaged in monitoring their own progress on the goals and each activity in the group ensuring transparency (see **Figure 2**).

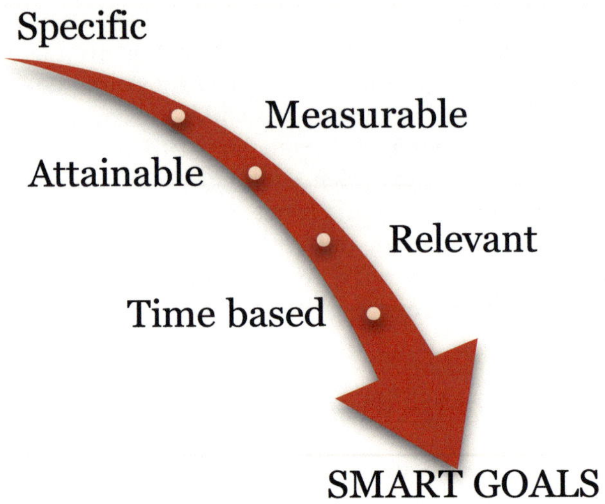

Figure 1.
Setting SMART goals in ACGs.

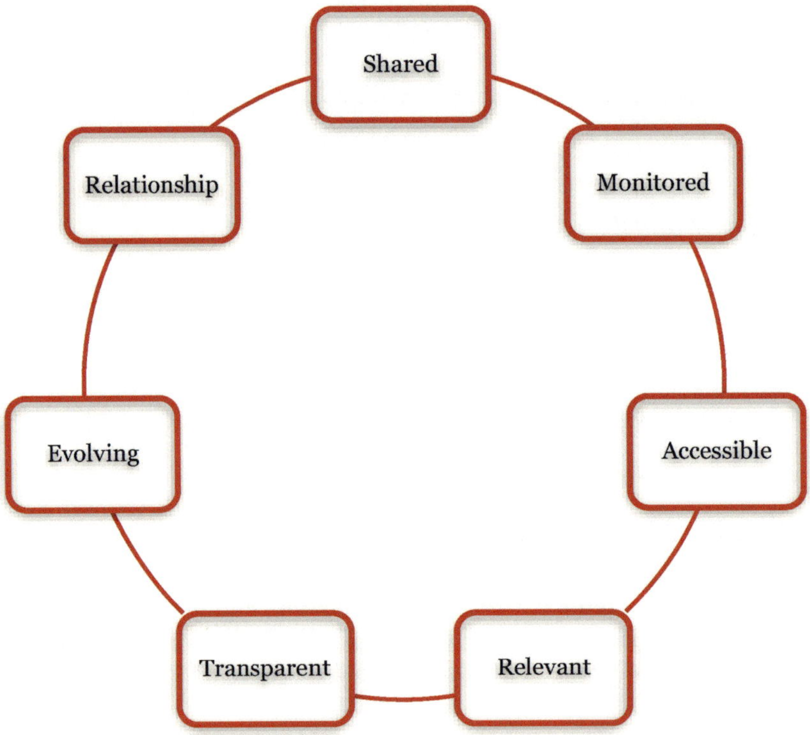

Figure 2.
The SMARTER framework based on Hersh et al. [41].

All goals are relevant to the person with aphasia, and care is provided in a way that builds rapport within the group. Personalized and qualitative therapeutic objectives enable group members to gain more insight into their communication barriers, individually and within the group.

For ACGs to achieve a SMARTER goal setting, the facilitator must read through the framework extensively and then answer the questions for each domain reported below in **Table 1** c.

	YES	NO
Shared		
• Has the person with aphasia and their family been able to prepare before attending the session?		
• Have family members, carers, and significant others been involved in goal setting?		
• Has the information been presented in a comprehensible way?		
• Is the information relevant to the person with aphasia?		
• Is the relationship between group members a trusting and collaborative one?		
• Have all people involved in goal setting understood the purpose of the procedure?		
• Have all people involved been able to express their individual needs and personal expectations?		
Relationship-Centered		
• Have the established goals been client-centered?		
• Has good rapport and trust been developed between the group members and facilitators?		
Relevant		
• Do the goals take into account the client's everyday life?		
• Have the client's family members and carers been involved in the goal-setting process?		
Accessible		
• Are goals written in an accessible aphasia-friendly format?		
• Can extra support be provided to ensure understanding?		
• Do PWA understand that they can change their goals if they wish to?		
Transparent		
• Are PWA and their carers aware of which goals will be worked on and how these will be assessed?		
• Is it clear how their personalized goals and the processes used to achieve these are linked?		
• Have they been able to assess what they will learn about during the group based on their current needs and goals?		
Monitored		
• Have the goals been written in a way that allows for ongoing evaluation?		
• Have the goals been written in a way that allows modifications?		
• Can these goals be used to review improvements or no improvements?		
Evolving		
• Are PWA and their carers aware that they can review the goals?		
• Are PWA and their carers aware that they can change the focus of the activities if they like?		

Table 1.
Specific questions involved in SMARTER goal setting framework as adapted from Hersh et al. [41].

4. The communication buddy system

A communication buddy is a communication and conversation partner assigned for each person with aphasia within the group. Their main goal is to facilitate the understanding and output (not necessarily verbal) for PWA within the group. Communication buddies should establish mutual support, promote learning about aphasia, facilitate communication, and promote communication skills enhancement [21]. Pairing in groups is based on Bion's theory of "containment" or "container and contained." According to Bion, the *theory of containment* is the capacity

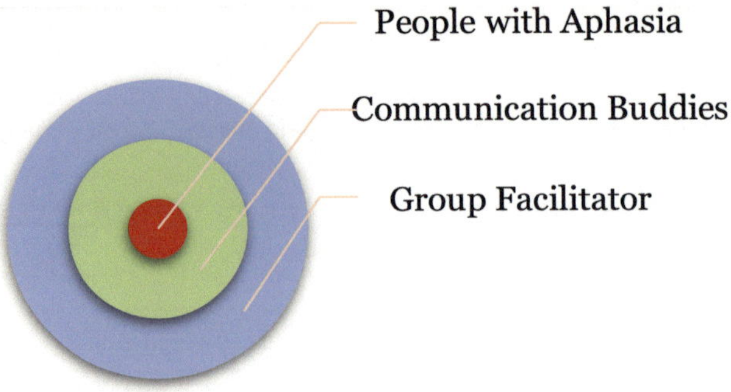

Figure 3.
The "essential" people that makeup ACGs.

of one individual to receive in himself/herself projections from another individual, which he/she then can sense and use as communications (from him/her), transform them, and finally give them back (or convey back) to the subject in a modified form (see **Figure 3**) [42].

Communication buddies can be:

- health care professionals.
- allied health rehabilitation students, e.g., speech and language therapy students.
- the client's carer, a family member, or friend.
- volunteers from aphasia and stroke support organizations.

Communication buddies should be identified and assigned by the person with aphasia or by the setting where the group is taking place, e.g., students in a university setting. Communication access, social contact, and active participation are crucial elements in aphasia group work. The person with aphasia, the group facilitator, and the communication buddy must collaborate to find the means and strategies that are most useful for the particular client during communication breakdowns. These may include gestures, drawing, picture support, simplified text, writing keywords, clarification statements, verification questions, eliminating environmental distractors, and summarizing (see **Table 2**). It is mandatory to work closely as a team to identify and tailor these strategies to the person with aphasia.

Means and strategies	Description
Gestures	Hand and body movements to express a meaning
Drawing	A picture or a diagram to represent a word or a meaning
Picture support	The use of a picture that can support understanding of the topic
Simplified text	A process to simplify a written message's content by paraphrasing
Writing keywords	The use of important/concept words to promote understanding
Clarification statements	To explain something in more detail to clarify the meaning
Verification questions	To ask yes/no or simple questions to confirm understanding
Environmental distractors	Things in the environment that move, make noise, or vibrate
Summarizing	To give a brief statement of the main points

Table 2.
The means and strategies for communication recovery.

4.1 Communication partners training

It is crucial that communication buddies, before their involvement with the group [41]:

- receive *education* on group therapy principles.
- *practice* scenarios via role-play and home assignments.
- watch videos and work on communication repair (i.e., how to modify, repeat or revise a message when the first communication attempt has failed) and facilitation strategies (i.e., active listening, good preparation, prompting, visual and verbal cues).
- receive *training* on feedback techniques, problem-solving, conversation skills, and self-reflection.

It is mandatory that communication partners learn how to implement the communication strategies within the group, communicate their message in simplified and accessible ways and assist the person with aphasia to get their message across [43].

5. Peer-led aphasia communication groups

Peer-led support groups for PWA are run by a person with aphasia and/or family member, with the assistance of their communication buddies, which aim to increase social interaction and peer support [44]. Peer-led models in aphasia communication groups provide access to constant peer support and may address some of the limitations of professionally-led support groups that may use formal agendas and have a strict group structure [45].

Studies examining peer-led support groups in other chronic conditions, that is, cancer survivors, have shown peer-led support groups (72.1%) are greater in the community than professionally led support groups (27.9%) [46], and there is a larger preference for peer than professional health care leaders [47]. For example, by reducing professional resources and interventions, peer-led ACGs can provide extensive, long-term opportunities for functional communication, social contact, friendship, and peer support [48]. Aphasia Connect has successfully expanded the range of services available for PWA across the UK by utilizing PWA as service providers (group leaders) as well as receivers (group members) [49]. Additionally, members of peer-led ACGs share a greater sense of empowerment and ownership as they provide *and* receive support [45]. In most UK aphasia peer-led groups, PWA receive training and ongoing support from speech-language therapists and trained volunteers to co-facilitate and codesign support groups [48]. Similarly, in other community-based ACGs such as Speakability UK, professional facilitators support the initial development of self-assisted groups for PWA, for example by suggesting resources and tips, and provide additional support upon request from group members [47].

Tregea and Brown [45] found that the features that are important for the successful functioning of a peer-led aphasia support group are:

- *Friendship*: instant bonds, feelings of belonging, and close friendships that resulted from shared experiences and mutual understanding.
- *Informality*: the sense of casualness, a relaxed environment with no pressure to communicate, and no formal agenda.

- *A supportive communication environment*: mutual support to participate, the need for patience, and encouragement to communicate.
- *Providing support*: a support base for PWA and their families to feel accepted, provision of resources, and information about aphasia.

Additional factors that facilitated peer leaders to start and run groups include informational support, practical support, attracting new members, time, venue and organization, and a pleasant communicative personality [45].

6. The role of the facilitator

Aphasia communication group facilitators should not necessarily be qualified SLTs but individuals who have been trained by professional SLTs and/or the research team, in case the group is part of a randomized controlled trial (RCT), ahead of the intervention or trial, with a particular focus on meaningful and effective communication with PWA [49]. Facilitators should be provided the National Aphasia Guidelines [50] for communication with PWA and be trained on partner conversation skills [43]. Facilitators should assist PWA to co-facilitate the group, and complete checklists at the end of each group session to evaluate fidelity to group content [49]. In a recent pilot feasibility RCT by Tarrant et al. [51] examining group signing intervention in PWA, the facilitators identified several benefits that they attributed to the intervention, starting with the prospect for PWA to meet peers and share personal experiences and the development of warm, empathetic friendships.

In contemporary clinical aphasiology, facilitated conversation in aphasia communication groups is a popular exercise but only a small number of published studies have documented how interactions occur in such group settings [51, 52]. One aspect of ACGs that has been mentioned in the recent literature, but that has not yet been the focus of intensive study, is participation management [51]. Facilitators report that finding ways to help people with limited expressive language participate in the conversation and the group, in general, is one of the central challenges faced by the clinicians and volunteers who lead these groups [51–53].

The study of Archer and colleagues [52] documents common approaches to assisting PWA to participate meaningfully within the group discussions. Results revealed a set of conversational practices used by facilitators and by group members with verbal output difficulties. Archer et al. [52] stated that "these practices took the form of two sequences viz. floor transfers and question-answer series" (p. 15). The identified sequences contributed to promoting meaningful conversational participation by group members with non-fluent aphasia.

After a national survey of third sector ACGs facilitators in the UK by VandenBerg et al. ([54], p. 25), results revealed that the factors described as important to supporting members' attendance in aphasia support groups were as follows:

- A kind induction (29%);
- Members' confidence in their communication skills (24%); and.
- Positive group dynamics (23%).

Also, in the same study ([54], p. 25), facilitators indicated that motivators for PWA's attendance were prioritized by their communication needs:

- "To get better at communicating" (16%);

- "To feel confident talking" (13%);
- "Meeting other people with aphasia" (18%).
- "Over peer support" (10%).
- or "Emotional support" (8%).

7. Evaluating the benefits of aphasia communication groups

Aphasia communication groups offer many advantages over traditional individual therapy models in the chronic stage [55]:

- *Provides naturalistic communication opportunities and practice*: the group setting facilitates provides a safe nonjudgmental environment for participants to practice and improve pragmatic skills, such as turn-taking, topic initiation, and maintenance [56]. Conversation practice and the use of spontaneous utterances may assist with the generalization of language skills to everyday interactions rather than the use of overlearned therapy targets [57].
- *Is cost-effective:* the session cost for each individual member can be reduced while maintaining a per-hour reimbursement that is similar to one-to-one session.
- *Has positive psycho-social outcomes*: PWA experience social isolation and reduced meaningful social engagements [42].

Group evaluation has three fundamental purposes [57]:

1. *To validate* and gain approval and acceptance of the status of the group. This process gains justification both for the choice of activities of the group and the continuing of its actions.
2. *To improve* by recognizing the importance of identifying any weak areas and how to improve these.
3. *To condemn* the weak practices of the group and to highlight the group's inadequacies.

To proceed with an evaluation process of the ACG, one could choose to evaluate all or any of the following areas [19]:

- *The process*: How were activities prepared and conducted? How was the method processed from the formation of the group to disbandment?
- *The members*: How did the members perform, either as individuals or within the group?
- *The resources*: Was the allocated venue, resources, room equipment, and time allocated sufficient?
- *The organization*: Did the group structure, context, content, and communication strategies, hinder or promote members' involvement?

- The objectives: Were the goals appropriate to the needs of the group? Were the goals sufficiently adapted to the individual needs of the group members?

8. The Aphasia Communication Team (TACT): a university-affiliated aphasia communication group

The TACT is a university-affiliated ACG in the Republic of Cyprus. The number of strokes in Cyprus range between 1200 and 1400 yearly [58]. If one considers a third of all stroke survivors have aphasia, this means, there are roughly 400 new cases of aphasia each year. About 61% continue to experience communication problems 1 year after stroke leading to fewer friendships and smaller social networks [59]. In the exploration of all the above factors influenced by aphasia, the idea of The Aphasia Communication Team – TACT emerged. TACT delivers benefits to PWA, families, and speech-language therapy trainees. TACT aims to provide stroke survivors support for learning and communication opportunities to promote living well with aphasia. TACT works on the barriers (areas of weakness of the person with aphasia and conversation partners that make communication difficult) and on what communication tools members could use to improve communication. TACT has a broad outlook for living well with aphasia and improving quality of life. Another goal targeted is the understanding that aphasia can be a long-term condition and that aphasia is a "family issue"—not just for the person with aphasia [60]. TACT promotes full participation and engagement in activities of interest. TACT encourages a safe, positive, environment, and is inclusive to all.

The Cyprus Stroke Association recruits stroke survivors and TACT is held at the premises of the Rehabilitation Clinic of the Cyprus University of Technology once a week, for 2 hours. Two groups have been established so far, with five stroke survivors with chronic aphasia and five communication buddies, for each group. Communication buddies are speech and language therapy students who serve as communication facilitators of each group member. The groups are supervised and coordinated by academic and scientific staff from the Department of Rehabilitation Sciences.

The Inclusion Criteria for participating in TACT is that PWA:

1. are discharged from formal rehabilitation [53].

2. have terminated individual speech and language therapy sessions [34].

3. aphasia is a predominant communication difficulty in relation to possible apraxia of speech or dysarthric symptoms [20].

4. can sustain approximately 2-hour participation with the group.

5. present with different severities of aphasia [18].

6. do not need additional medical support while being at group [55].

7. should manage toileting or have additional support from a carer [34].

8. have given written consent to participate and sign a confidentiality contract with the clinic and CSA.

Group members are assessed on psychometric measures (language, cognition, and quality of life) at the beginning and the end of each block of therapy. Therapy consists of a 12-week block of weekly sessions. The assessment procedure is based on the

International Population Registry for Aphasia after Stroke (I-PRAISE) protocol [61] in combination with Attard et al's. [53] ICF-based assessment protocol. This is deemed necessary to measure improvement or change in behaviors post-therapy (see **Table 3**).

Group members are encouraged to share experiences by using technology and tablets. They also practice total communication skills, i.e., adding gestures, drawing, and writing to speech. The main topics of discussion are acquiring new knowledge on stroke and aphasia, linking the data to members' personal experiences, clarifying questions and misunderstandings about their condition, and sharing stories about their life before stroke, the incidence itself, and living with aphasia (see **Figure 4**).

Group member's outcomes consist of change or improvement in measures of functional communication, the overall severity of language impairment, auditory comprehension, spoken language (including naming), reading, and writing from

ICF domain-outcome measures	
Aphasia impairment	• Aphasia Severity Rating Scale; ASRS by the shortened version of the Boston Diagnostic Aphasia Examination; BDAE • Western Aphasia Battery–Revised Aphasia Quotient; WAB–R AQ
Activity & participation	• Amsterdam Nijmegen Everyday Language Test; ANELT • Scenario Test • Communicative Effectiveness Index; CETI
Contextual Factors	• Therapy Outcome Measure; TOM • Subjective Index of Physical and Social Outcome; SIPSO
Quality of life	• Stroke and Aphasia Quality of Life Score; SAQOL-39 g • Assessment of Living with Aphasia; ALA
Psychological health	• General Health Questionnaire-12; GHQ-12 • Perception of Patient-Centeredness/Consultation Care Measure

Table 3.
ACGs outcome measures.

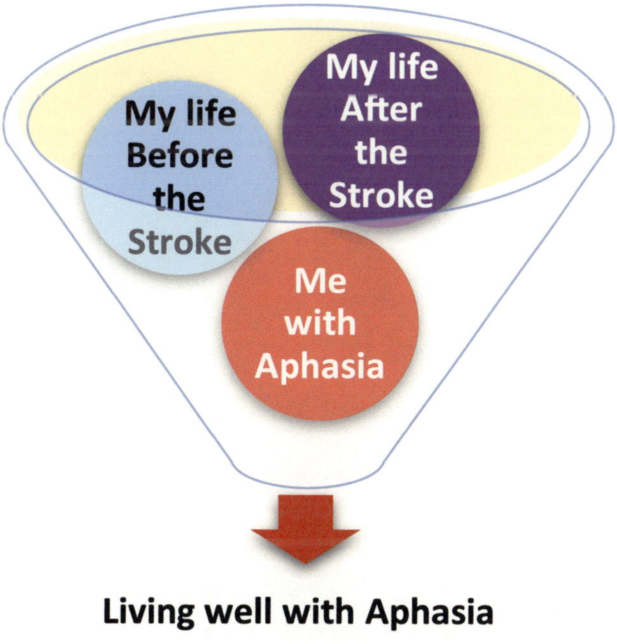

Figure 4.
The main conversation "topics" for TACT members.

baseline, overall communication self-rating, and quality of life after stroke. Data gathered via assessment procedures are digitalized for each individual member on a database using the RELEASE protocol [61]. The use of the communication buddy system, the involvement of the total communication approach, the systematic assessment, and the collection of individual patient data (IPD) sets enable the TACT team to measure the effectiveness and efficacy of group therapy interventions for people with chronic aphasia in terms of use of functional communication, social inclusion [14], and quality of life [31].

9. Conclusion

There is no doubt that Aphasia Communication Groups (ACGs) are of great benefit for people with chronic aphasia. ACGs are associated overall with improvement in communication, social networks, and community access. To achieve this, ACGs facilitators, participating members, and communication buddies should have equal involvement in the realization of the group.

Conflict of interest

The authors declare no conflict of interest.

Author details

Marina Charalambous[1,2] and Maria Kambanaros[1*]

1 Rehabilitation Sciences Department, Cyprus University of Technology, Limassol, Cyprus

2 Laboratory of Cognitive and Neurological Sciences, University of Fribourg, Switzerland

*Address all correspondence to: maria.kambanaros@cut.ac.cy

References

[1] Mitchell C, Gittins M, Tyson SF, Vail A, Conroy P, Paley L, et al. Prevalence of aphasia and dysarthria among inpatient stroke survivors: Describing the population, therapy provision and outcomes on discharge. Aphasiology. 2020;**4**:1-11

[2] Berg K, Isaksen J, Wallace S, Cruice M, Simmons-Mackie N, Worrall L. Establishing consensus on a definition of aphasia: An e-Delphi study of international aphasia researchers. Aphasiology. 2020:1-16. DOI:10.1080/02687038.2020.1852003

[3] Ali M, Lyden P, Brady M, VISTA Collaboration. Aphasia and dysarthria in acute stroke: Recovery and functional outcome. International Journal of Stroke. 2015;**10**(3):400-406

[4] Burfein P, Roxbury T, de Silva N, Copland D. Return to work for stroke survivors with aphasia: Preliminary findings of a scoping review. In: The Inaugural Herston Health Precinct Symposium, 7-11 Dec 2020. Royal Brisbane and: Women's Hospital; 2016

[5] Manning M, MacFarlane A, Hickey A, Franklin S. Perspectives of people with aphasia post-stroke towards personal recovery and living successfully: A systematic review and thematic synthesis. PLoS One. 2019; **14**(3):e0214200

[6] Laures-Gore JS, Dotson VM, Belagaje S. Depression in poststroke aphasia. American Journal of Speech-Language Pathology. 2020;**29**(4): 1798-1810

[7] Hoover E, McFee A, DeDe G. Efficacy of group conversation intervention in individuals with severe profiles of aphasia. Seminars in Speech and Language. 2020;**41**(1):71-82

[8] Doedens W, Meteyard L. Measures of functional, real-world communication for aphasia: A critical review. Aphasiology. 2020;**34**(4):492-514

[9] Azios JH, Strong KA, Archer B, Douglas NF, Simmons-Mackie N, Worrall L. Friendship matters: A research agenda for aphasia. Aphasiology. 2021:1-20. DOI: 10.1080/02687038.2021.1873908

[10] Koleck M, Gana K, Lucot C, Darrigrand B, Mazaux JM, Glize B. Quality of life in aphasic patients 1 year after a first stroke. Quality of Life Research. 2017;**26**(1):45-54

[11] Tippett DC, Hillis AE. Where are aphasia theory and management "headed". F1000 Research. 2017;**6**:6

[12] Harmon TG, Lin ML, Scronce G, Jacks A. Supporting confidence and participation for people with aphasia through student interaction: A descriptive study on the effects of an interdisciplinary campus program. Journal of Allied Health. 2019;**48**(4): e107-e112

[13] Lee JB, Azios JH. Facilitator behaviors leading to engagement and disengagement in aphasia conversation groups. American Journal of Speech-Language Pathology. 2020;**29**(1S): 393-411

[14] World Health Organization. International Classification for Functioning, Disability and Health (ICF): Short Version. Geneva, Switzerland: World Health Organization; 2001

[15] LPAA Project Group, Chapey R, Duchan J, Elman R, Garcia L, Lyon JG, et al. Life participation approach to aphasia: A statement of values for the future. In: Chapey R, editor. Language Intervention Strategies in Aphasia and Related Neurogenic Communication Disorders. Baltimore, MD: Lippincott Williams & Wilkins; 2001. pp. 279-289

[16] Pettigrove K. Scoping review protocol: Characteristics and impacts of community aphasia group facilitation. Disability and Rehabilitation. 2020. DOI: 10.13140/RG.2.2.13592.01285

[17] Elman RJ. Introduction to group treatment of neurogenic communication disorders. In: Elman RJ, editor. Group Treatment of Neurogenic Communication Disorders: The Expert Clinician's Approach. 2nd ed. San Diego: Plural Publishing, Inc.; 2007

[18] Elman RJ, Bernstein-Ellis E. The efficacy of group communication treatment in adults with chronic aphasia. Journal of Speech, Language, and Hearing Research. 1999;**42**(2): 411-419

[19] Elwyn G, Macfarlane F, Greenhalgh T. Groups: A Guide to Small Group Work in Healthcare, Management, Education and Research. 1st ed. Oxon: CRC Press; 2001. DOI: 10.1201/9781315384375

[20] Elman RJ. Group Treatment of Neurogenic Communication Disorders: The Expert Clinician's Approach. 2nd ed. Plural Pub: San Diego (CA); 2007

[21] Charalambous M, Kambanaros M. Aphasia communication groups in Cyprus: The Aphasia Communication Team (TACT). Joined e-Conference of the European Stroke Organization (ESO) and the World Stroke Organization (WSO). International Journal of Stroke. 2020;**15**(Suppl. 1): 724-724

[22] Bronken BA, Kirkevold M, Martinsen R, Kvigne K. The aphasic storyteller: Coconstructing stories to promote psychosocial well-being after stroke. Qualitative Health Research. 2012;**22**(10):1303-1316

[23] Kambanaros M. Evaluating personal stroke narratives from bilingual Greek-English immigrants with aphasia. Folia Phoniatrica et Logopaedica. 2019; **71**(2-3):101-115

[24] Cruice M, Aujla S, Bannister S, Botting N, Boyle M, Charles N, et al. Creating a novel approach to discourse treatment through coproduction with people with aphasia and speech and language therapists. Aphasiology. 2021:1-23. DOI: 10.1080/02687038.2021.1942775

[25] Fama ME, Baron CR, Hatfield B, Turkeltaub PE. Group therapy as a social context for aphasia recovery: A pilot, observational study in an acute rehabilitation hospital. Topics in Stroke Rehabilitation. 2016;**23**(4):276-283

[26] Worall L. The Seven Habits of highly effective aphasia therapists: The perspective of people living with aphasia. International Journal of Speech-Language Pathology. 2019;**21**(5):438-447. DOI: 10.1080/17549507.2019.1660804

[27] Royal College of Speech and Language Therapists. The Five Good Communication Standards. London, UK: Royal College of Speech and Language Therapists; 2016

[28] Lanyon L, Worrall L, Rose M. "It's not really worth my while": Understanding contextual factors contributing to decisions to participate in community aphasia groups. Disability and Rehabilitation. 2019;**41**(9): 1024-1036

[29] Simmons-Mackie N, Savage MC, Worrall L. Conversation therapy for aphasia: A qualitative review of the literature. International Journal of Language & Communication Disorders. 2014;**49**(5):511-526

[30] Attard M, Lanyon L, Togher L, Rose M. Consumer perspectives on community aphasia groups: A narrative literature review in the context of psychological well-being. Aphasiology. 2015;**29**(8):983-1019

[31] Lanyon L, Worrall L, Rose M. What really matters to people with aphasia when it comes to group work? A qualitative investigation of factors impacting participation and integration. International Journal of Language & Communication Disorders. 2018; **53**(3):526-541

[32] Charalambous M, Kambanaros M, Annoni JM. Are people with aphasia (PWA) involved in the creation of quality of life and aphasia impact-related questionnaires? A scoping review. Brain Science. 2020;**10**(10):688

[33] Paul DR, Frattali CM, Holland AL, Thompson CK, Caperton CJ, Slater SC. The American Speech-Language-Hearing Association Quality of Communication Life Scale (QCL): Manual. Rockville, MD, USA: American Speech-Language-Hearing Association; 2004

[34] Hunt J. Groups organizations. In: Managing People at Work (3e). New York: McCraw- Hill; 1992

[35] Hersh D. "From the Ground Up": The Talkback Group Program in South Australia. In: Elman RJ, editor. Group Treatment of Neurogenic Communication Disorders: The Expert Clinician's Approach. 2nd ed. San Diego: Plural Publishing, Inc.; 2007

[36] Wallace SE, Donoso EV, Saylor BA, Lapp E, Eskanderb J. Designing occupational therapy home programs for people with aphasia: Aphasia-friendly modifications. Perspectives of the ASHA Special Interest Groups. 2020;**5**:425-434

[37] Rose ML, Attard MC. Practices and challenges in community aphasia groups in Australia: Results of a national survey. International Journal of Speech-Language Pathology. 2015;**17**(3):241-251

[38] Pitt R, Theodoros D, Hill AJ, Russell T. The development and feasibility of an online aphasia group intervention and networking program - TeleGAIN. International Journal of Speech-Language Pathology. 2019;**21**(1):23-36

[39] Pitt R, Theodoros D, Hill AJ, Russell T. The impact of the telerehabilitation group aphasia intervention and networking programme on communication, participation, and quality of life in people with aphasia. International Journal of Speech-Language Pathology. 2019;**21**(5):513-523

[40] Worrall L, Sherratt S, Rogers P, Howe T, Hersh D, Ferguson A, et al. What people with aphasia want: Their goals according to the ICF. Aphasiology. 2011;**25**(3):309-322

[41] Hersh D, Worrall L, Howe T, Sherratt S, Davidson B. SMARTER goal setting in aphasia rehabilitation. Aphasiology. 2012;**26**(2):220-233

[42] Bion W. Experiences in Groups and Other Papers. London: William Heinemann; 1961

[43] Mueller AI. The effects of communication partner training on people with aphasia and their communication partners. Speech-Language Pathology Posters. Department of Communication Disorders and Deaf Education. Missouri, USA: Fontbonne University; 2020;**10**:1

[44] Simmons-Mackie N, Raymer A, Cherney LR. Communication partner training in aphasia: An updated systematic review. Archives of Physical Medicine and Rehabilitation. 2016;**97**(12):2202-2221.e8

[45] Tregea S, Brown K. What makes a successful peer-led aphasia support group? Aphasiology. 2013;**27**(5):581-598

[46] Stevinson C, Lydon A, Amir Z. Characteristics of professionally-led and

peer-led cancer support groups in the United Kingdom. Journal of Cancer Survivorship. 2010;**4**(4):331-338

[47] Butow PN, Kirsten LT, Ussher JM, Wain GV, Sandoval M, Hobbs KM, et al. What is the ideal support group? Views of Australian people with cancer and their carers. Psycho-Oncology. Netherlands: Elsevier; 2007;**16**(11):1039-1045

[48] Code C, Eales C, Pearl G, Conan M, Cowin K, Hickin J. Supported self-help groups for aphasic people. In: The Sciences of Aphasia. 2003. pp. 187-200. DOI: 10.1016/B978-008044073-6/50014-6

[49] Pound C, Duchan J, Penman T, Hewitt A, Parr S. Communication access to organisations: Inclusionary practices for people with aphasia. Aphasiology. 2007;**21**(1):23-38

[50] National Health and Medical Research Council (NHMRC) Centre for Clinical Research Excellence (CCRE) in Aphasia Rehabilitation. Australian Aphasia Rehabilitation Pathway (AARP). 2014. Available from: http://www.aphasiapathway.com.au [Retrieved: 7 June 2021]

[51] Tarrant M, Carter M, Dean SG, Taylor R, Warren FC, Spencer A, et al. Singing for people with aphasia (SPA): Results of a pilot feasibility randomised controlled trial of a group singing intervention investigating acceptability and feasibility. BMJ Open. 2021;**11**(1):e040544

[52] Archer B, Azios JH, Gulick N, Tetnowski J. Facilitating participation in conversation groups for aphasia. Aphasiology. 2020;**35**:1-19

[53] Attard MC, Loupis Y, Togher L, Rose ML. The efficacy of an inter-disciplinary community aphasia group for living well with aphasia. Aphasiology. 2018;**32**(2):105-138

[54] Vanden Berg K, Ali M, Cruice M, Brady MC. Support groups for people with aphasia: A national survey of third sector group facilitators in the UK. Aphasiology. 2018;**32**(Supp. 1):233-236. DOI: 10.1080/02687038.2018.1487016

[55] Layfield CA, Ballard KJ, Robin DA. Evaluating group therapy for aphasia: What is the evidence? EBP Briefs. 2013;**7**(5):1-17. [Bloomington, MN: Pearson]

[56] Elman RJ. The importance of aphasia group treatment for rebuilding community and health. Topics in Language Disorders. 2007;**27**(4): 300-308

[57] Breakwell G, Millard L. Basic Evaluation Methods: Analysing Performance, Procedure and Practice. Leicester: British Phycologist Society; 1995

[58] Norrving B, Barrick J, Davalos A, Dichgans M, Cordonnier C, Guekht A, et al. Action plan for stroke in Europe 2018-2030. European Stroke Journal. 2018;**3**(4):309-336

[59] Georgiou A, Konstantinou N, Phinikettos I, Kambanaros M. Neuronavigated theta burst stimulation for chronic aphasia: Two exploratory case studies. Clinical Linguistics & Phonetics. 2019;**33**(6):532-546

[60] Matos LM, Cruice M. Consequences of stroke and aphasia according to the ICF domains: Views of Portuguese people with aphasia, family members and professionals. Aphasiology. 2014;**28**(7):771-796

[61] Brady MC, Ali M, Vanden Berg K, Williams LJ, Williams LR, Abo M, et al. RELEASE: A protocol for a systematic review based, individual participant data, meta-and network meta-analysis, of complex speech-language therapy interventions for stroke-related aphasia. Aphasiology. 2020;**34**(2):137-157